Conversations With My Healers

CONVERSATIONS WITH MY HEALERS

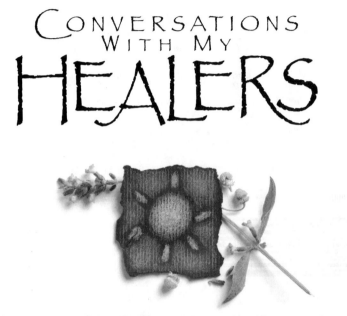

MY JOURNEY TO WELLNESS
FROM BREAST CANCER

by Cynthia Ploski

COUNCIL OAK PUBLISHING
TULSA, OKLAHOMA

Nothing in this book should be construed by the
reader as medical advice. Both author and publisher strongly recommend
regular medical check-ups. Should you find yourself in need of treatment, the
advice of your own physician should be followed.

Council Oak Books, Tulsa, OK 74120
©1995 Cynthia Ploski. All rights reserved
99 98 97 96 95   5 4 3 2 1
ISBN 1-57178-010-6
Cover and book designed by Carol Stanton

Library of Congress Cataloging-in-Publication Data

Ploski, Cynthia, 1932–
      Conversations with my healers : my journey to wellness from breast
cancer /Cynthia Ploski.
          p.   cm.
      Includes bibliographical references.
      ISBN 1-57178-010-6 (cloth)
      1. Ploski, Cynthia, 1932- – Health.   2. Breast–Cancer–Patients–
United States—Biography. 3. Breast–Cancer–Alternative treatment
I. Title.
RC280.B8P56   1995
362.1'9699449'0092—dc20
      [B]   95-11792
                                                                   CIP

In honor of the mother of us all
who answered my call

Contents

A Note to the Reader

This story is a true one, at times painful, at times exalting; but always leading me forward. I say without reservation, it has been the most profound experience of my life.

From such experience comes knowledge, and from knowledge comes strength. Adventures along the road to recovery were my teachers, and I hope that my experiences will be empowering to you, esteemed reader, to whom I offer this work.

As you will see, I availed myself of many therapies, both traditional and non-traditional. Please be aware, however, that what I write about does not constitute, nor substitute for, medical advice.

Each person has a different path to follow, and must make choices based on his or her best judgement. You must evaluate information from a wide variety of sources and seek medical advice from your health care provider.

No two cases are alike. Therapies that were helpful to me may not necessarily be helpful to you. This book is not a "how to" manual. It is simply the story of my personal journey back to wellness, which I desire to share with you—because all of us, healthy or well, have a lot in common as human beings in this great adventure called living.

Acknowledgments

Along my path, many people have reached out to help me. I could never name them all to thank them, for they number in the thousands, seen and unseen.

But I would like to thank a few who have been especially close to me:

My dear husband, Ted Ploski, unfailingly supportive, even in the darkest times;

My beloved children: Melanie Kurtz, Jim Berresse, Alissa Finley, Michael Berresse, and their families, whose love transcended the miles of separation;

My remarkable mother, Anne Feindel, whose affirmations and prayers got all of Heaven involved;

My special friends, Mary Carroll Nelson and Betty Rice, who activated the network of healing and saw to my physical and spiritual needs;

And my publisher, Sally Dennison of Council Oak Books, who believed this material needed to be set forth.

I am truly grateful to you all.

Introduction

We are indeed living in a turbulent world of change. We have come face to face with the realities of war. Not the war of nation against nation but the war against pollution, poverty, destruction of natural resources and disease. AIDS is frightening in its apparently uncheckable spread and the shadow of death; cancer has reached a point where one out of three people in the United States will contract it in some form. Breast cancer in New Mexico escalated from one in twenty in 1972 to one in eight by 1995.

In the war against cancer, many disciplines unite to fight the enemy. There are the armies of allopathic medicine: surgery, chemotherapy, radiation, drugs and research. These forces generate and spend huge amounts of money. They represent deeply vested interests with formidable power on every level, from patient to government. They have made significant progress in the treatment of cancer and should be considered as a means of treatment by anyone who has contracted the disease.

There are other ways to fight cancer, however, that also have significant value. These disciplines are holistic in nature, stemming from a belief that true healing must consider the needs of not only the body but the mind and soul as well. Many of these traditions such as acupuncture, Chinese herbal medicine and Ayurvedic medicine have been used for at least four thousand years. As long as there have been people there have been shamans and others who heal by faith or laying on of hands. It has been the recent fashion to regard these disciplines as quackery; yet there is a current upswelling of interest on the part of ordinary people who wish to take a more active part in their own healing.

Perhaps because of this escalation of interest, our ability to choose is being threatened. In the name of protecting the people, powerful lobbies are attempting to regulate the sale of herbal medicines and nutritional supplements. The entire health care system is in acute transition.

Against this backdrop I am presenting my own experience. I feel that people should know the choices available to them and move from being passive "patients" to being active co-practitioners in their own healing.

I chose to undergo the traditional allopathic treatments for breast cancer—surgery, chemotherapy and radiation therapy. I also chose to use acupuncture, nutrition, shamanism, transpersonal counseling, herbs and naturopathy to round out the allopathic treatment and support me through it.

In these chapters I will tell you how a mastectomy is performed and its results in my body. I will give you information about the effects of chemotherapy and radiation from the point of view of my own experience. You will know how acupuncture feels, and what it did for me; how I experience the laying on of hands and shaman's journey; what color therapy is all about, and more. Each healer will add to my story through conversations.

I am not the same person I was five years ago. Being diagnosed and treated for breast cancer opened the door for a profound encounter with myself and my mortality that became a transformational journey. No longer am I the woman who danced slowly through life blanketed in normalcy. Through this rite of passage I have become truly alive. It sounds crazy to see breast cancer as a blessing, but it really has been so. Of course there have been pain and fear and horror, but encountering them has moved me through this gauntlet into a new existence. Cancer became my rebirth canal.

I did not make this journey alone. Along the way my healers materialized, each one contributing his or her special skills to help me become whole. I did find out that wholeness does not necessarily mean having all your body parts. Wholeness is a state of body/mind/soul.

There have been many healers in my journey. The ones who helped me professionally are featured in this manuscript. But there are many others, seen and unseen, from my beloved family and friends to those only approached through meditation and prayer. They were there for me, and I will always be appreciative.

Although this is my deeply personal narrative I am putting it forth in the belief that my experiences will give hope to others who are facing the same challenges. We are a mighty sisterhood. We can make this journey hand in hand.

My Journey Begins

W   I   L   L   I   A   M   J   .   M   C   I   V   E   R

The Surgeon

This isn't me. This is some kind of bad dream! I was floating in a strange sense of unreality. It swept me away from the crashing wave of fear which nearly drowned out Dr. McIver's words as he told Ted and me the bad news about my biopsy.

But then my stomach tightened with dread as the real world slowly brought me back. With great kindness and compassion Dr. McIver explained the next steps. The lump had not been a tumor, rather a group of cancerous lymph nodes that had grown together. The primary tumor had to be located, so he set up an appointment with a radiologist for more detailed mammograms. Deeply shaken, we left the office holding hands. "We'll beat this together," my husband murmured as he hugged me in the car. His voice was husky and there were tears in his eyes. There were tears in my eyes also, but I was too dazed to weep.

It had begun six months earlier, with a call from my gynecologist. The routine mammogram had been normal, but there was an enlargement of lymph glands that needed to be checked. At his office he could feel no lump, and he decided that maybe the lymph nodes had enlarged to fight a previous skin irritation in the armpit. It was not until four months later, on a trip through New England, that—as I crossed my arms in the back seat of the car—I felt a lump in my right breast. I called the gynecologist when I got home and this time he referred me to Dr. McIver, an Albuquerque surgeon specializing in breast care.

Looking back, I realize I should have been referred for a biopsy immediately after the mammogram. We are conditioned to have total faith in doctors' ability to take care of us. When the doctor in effect dismissed the mammogram report, I thought he knew best. Or maybe fear made me want to believe him. Had it been checked out right away, perhaps the cancer would have not spread as far. My treatment might have been less radical and my chances of survival better.

For me, it is past history, but I want to alert others. This is my impassioned plea: insist on checking out anything suspicious right away! Even if you are afraid. Especially if you are afraid. Don't let fear paralyze you. It is your own body and you are in charge of keeping it healthy, not anyone else.

Anyway, despite Dr. McIver's assurances that most lumps are benign, fear shot my blood pressure so high that the outpatient surgery clinic refused to proceed with the biopsy. I went home to go on medication and try again. Two weeks later I returned, and this time Dr. McIver was able to operate. I was given some sort of analgesic, and although I could hear Dr. McIver and the nurses talking back and forth, I felt no pain. Ted had to pick up his sister Toni at the airport, so they released me in a short while, groggy and with a bunch of stitches, to the custody of my dear friend Betty Rice, who drove me home.

A few days later came the biopsy report in Dr. McIver's office, and so began a round of tests. First, the radiologist took many detailed pictures, located a suspicious area and confirmed the tumor by a sonogram. Can you believe we were relieved to find a tumor? At least it was something definite, not some mysterious, undefined cancer coursing through my body. It was small, and we thought, Good! Less likelihood that it has spread. We were wrong. Size doesn't always predict aggressiveness.

Then there were blood tests, chest x-rays and a whole body bone scan to see if the cancer had spread beyond the lymph system. To our relief, they were all negative. The bone scan involved being injected with a short-life radioactive substance which is taken up by the bones in a couple of hours, then about a half hour of lying still while a big camera moved over my body taking pictures. While this was going on I was mentally walking in my special imaginary garden, feeling the beauty of the plants and trees and meeting healers who were making me well. In actuality, I had just begun meeting my real healers—and you will meet them too, in these pages.

My feelings during this time of diagnosis? Just about every emotion you could imagine, except bliss. Anger that my body had betrayed me. I had no risk factors, I was always conscious of good nutrition and exercise, I was strong, I was healthy. I probably weighed fifteen pounds more than I should and I did like my evening glasses of wine, but this did not seem important in the whole scheme of things. My mother was still alive at ninety-two and her parents lived into their nineties also. I had great genes! So why did this sinister, evil thing creep into my body? Why had my body not fought it off?

Then there was depression, a feeling of powerlessness. I was a victim. All my hopes and plans might never come to fruition. Would I ever see my grandchildren grow up? Would I ever again be able to hike the mountains or roam the high mesa or hug the ponderosa pines, inhaling their glorious spicy fragrance? I love life! I love the people in my life! Would I have to give that up to a few years of pain and suffering, then leave it all behind?

Somewhere in the depths of that depression was born a germ of determination that led to an unconscious decision to fight. So I began to look for information, for shreds of hope, for other people's miracles, for positive energy anywhere I could find it. I bargained, I pleaded with God, and I put on my fighting armor and turned outward to find out why I had cancer and who could help me overcome it.

But all along my biggest battle was with my own fear. I would awaken each morning to a nightmare of living and go to sleep each night to some place where dreams became my comforting reality. I was afraid of death; I was afraid of pain; I was afraid of loss; I was afraid of the future; I was afraid of everything.

Fear is a normal reaction to threat, but my fear went beyond that. As I later began to explore my inner self, I found a lifetime of fear and anxiety to which I was so accustomed I didn't even recognize it. I am still sorting out its roots, but I have a strong remembrance of a little girl praying by her bed as she was taught:
"Now I lay me down to sleep
I pray the Lord my soul to keep.
If I should die before I wake,
I pray the Lord my soul to take."
And then that little girl in terror would awaken in the night and run crying to her mother's bed for comfort. There was no Catholic guardian angel to protect me. I couldn't even be sure I would wake up in the morning. These childhood fears got buried and forgotten, but still colored my life.

I remember as a young mother praying, imploring daily that my children would be kept safe and healthy—the same childhood fear transposed. And as for cancer, my mother cannot yet even say the word. She taught me not to sit on public toilet seats, never to kiss anyone on the mouth, to stay away from people with colds or strangers who might have colds, and always to wash my hands because of germs. I remember being concerned about every lump and bump on my body—not a hypochondriac, mind you, because I never said anything about it out loud. I just stuffed it inside and developed hypertension.

Now fear, my constant companion, had finally transformed into something tangible, and became my greatest battle. I found many ways to combat it, but it always came back, catching me unawares and vulnerable. Perhaps it always will, but I have learned to fight it with what I call "radical trust"—and that is a process of growth.

Meanwhile, a host of family and friends came to my assistance with loving thoughts and expressions of faith. This network of support and prayer has been a source of much healing energy, and I grieve for anyone who has to go through cancer alone. I would say to them, "Reach out. Locate a support group. Know that others share your journey and that you can help one another towards wellness." I have found it to be so.

At the end of a strange, formless pool of time, surgery day arrived. The day before, my friend Teresa had given me a hypnotherapy session during which she visualized the cancer leaving my body and flying off to the North. It relaxed me so that I could sleep that night, despite the anxiety of impending surgery.

Since I had chosen a modified radical mastectomy, before sleeping I said good-by to my breast. I remembered all the wonderful things it had done for me, the four healthy babies it had fed, the pleasure of loving caresses. I told it that losing its life would save mine, and thanked it for serving me so well. I knew there would be some work to do on my feminine self image, but I had already learned from a hysterectomy several years earlier that being a woman is far more than having all your body parts. You may lose a uterus or a breast but you are still you. It does not shatter wholeness. You are still yourself, a female, with two "X" chromosomes and the same womanly spirit.

So breakfastless and reasonably calm, Ted and I waded through the web of hospital admitting paperwork and, after a shower with germicidal soap, wearing a modish hospital gown and fashionable new plastic bracelet, I was ready to hold court for the visitors who had come to lend me their love and support.

My dear son Jim flew up from Phoenix to spend the day with me. Friends Betty, Teresa, Norma and Grace were there and husband Ted, of course. My sister-in-law Toni had extended her visit from Chicago to help nurse me when I returned home from the hospital, and she was on the home front offering support to my mother. How did the morning slide by? In a strange sense of unreality, like we were actors on a stage.

Finally a nurse gave me a pre-op shot which made my mouth feel like cotton and my attitude somewhat giddy. Teresa spent a little time with me alone, relaxing me and preparing me for the time my body would be in someone else's hands and my spirit waiting somewhere until it was over. Then my husband and my son and the entourage accompanied me on that great gurney ride where you watch the ceiling slide by until they close the elevator doors.

Next came the rustle and bustle of the operating room—mysterious masked figures moving around doing important things—bright lights—coolness—getting moved onto an operating table—a woman's voice saying "Count to ten"—a needle prick in the arm—One—two—and the next thing I know I am breathing cool oxygen and a voice is calling, "Cynthia, you're in the recovery room. Your surgery is all over." My body is totally relaxed, I feel no pain, just peace and gratitude that it is over, and surprise that it had all happened so quickly.

The full group was waiting for me in my room. Dr. McIver had met with Ted after the surgery and told him all went well and there was little bleeding. Later that afternoon the anesthesiologist came to my room. Did I remember her? Oh, yes, but she had worked so quickly I hadn't had a chance to do my little surrender routine. Perhaps I had not realized it, she told me, but she worked with me on "another level" preparing me for surgery. I thanked her, and felt glad there were people healing on all levels within the medical profession.

Teresa had a profound experience while I was in surgery. She left the hospital and was walking down the street when she saw the flash of a silvery object in the sky, emitting radiation. She sat on a curb and watched it hang motionless in the sky for about fifteen minutes, then disappear. Back in the hospital chapel, in prayer, she fell into a trance and was with me on that other level exchanging our black robes for white ones. The impression was we had passed through a crisis and were on the other side of it.

I was up and walking within a couple of hours after returning to my room. Although I was still attached to an intravenous drip, I just toddled along holding the drip tree beside me. With this kind of surgery there are no tubes in various orifices, so I was pretty comfortable—and if I felt pain I could press a button and send a dose of morphine into my I-V from a friendly machine at bedside. Bandages hid the stapled incision from my eyes, for which I was grateful. It was too soon to look at myself.

Two days later, feeling pretty good, having had little real pain, I went home. Reaching the top of the car window was impossible, but because the chest muscles were intact I had some mobility and use of the arm right away. There followed a week of being coddled and cared for by Ted and Toni.

Sometime during that week I met the challenge of looking at my body. My right side, reflected back to me in the bathroom mirror, was the chest of a boy, slashed into halves by an angry red horizontal incision from which hung two drains. The other side looked normal, giving me the odd sensation of being half male and half female. *Well, Cynthia, this is a strange state of affairs,* I thought, *but you are going to get used to it.*

Challenge met. I survived.

I spent a lot of time that week reading *Love, Medicine and Miracles* by Dr. Bernie Siegel. Bernie was good for my attitude, but nevertheless as the week progressed and the pathology report time drew nearer, I became a basket case. All my good intentions vanished. I was a mess.

Finally Dr. McIver called with the results. It wasn't good news. He had removed 23 lymph nodes, out of which 14 were contaminated with cancer, 9 were not. He said he saw no evidence that the cancer had spread beyond the axillary area—words I clung to—but that I would definitely need chemotherapy.

Anxiety turned into depression, and the full circle of emotional stuff and junk. But reason returned after I called a friend and fellow artist Marty Slaymaker, who recommended her oncologist, Dr. Saiki. Marty had a mastectomy something like eighteen years ago, and a recurrence of the cancer in 1984. She is a wonderful role model, and very active in a cancer support group. Through Dr. McIver's recommendation and Marty's intercession, Dr. Saiki agreed to take me on as a patient.

So I was to move along from surgery to chemotherapy, but Dr.

McIver assured me he was not through with me. "I'll be following you for the next twenty years," he stated, and those words were very welcome to my ears.

Twenty-two months later, as I walked into Dr. McIver's inner sanctum, I felt light, almost giggly. Every other visit had had a certain amount of dread attached, but this was not a checkup, it was an interview for my book. I felt like a different Cynthia from the woman who had her life blown apart there two years before. This altered me felt a new energy, a sense of purpose, health and vitality.

I settled into a soft chair in that very same room where we had heard the bad news. As I pulled out my tape recorder, reflections of earlier emotions flooded back—fear, more fear, sadness, hopelessness, anxiety—and a little bit of hope as I grabbed onto each faintly positive word my compassionate surgeon spoke.

Wouldn't it have been wonderful if I could have looked ahead to see myself coming back for this interview, a purified, reworked me? It might have saved a lot of suffering, but it would have been like flying from Los Angeles to Albuquerque without ever seeing the Grand Canyon, the Painted Desert, the Arizona mountains, the Indian reservations, the Meteor Crater or the Petrified Forest. I would have arrived at the destination, but would have missed the journey.

Dr. McIver's booming "Hello, Mrs. Ploski" and cordial handshake interrupted my reverie.

William J. McIver is a gentle giant of a man whose warm demeanor and hearty voice make patients feel comfortable immediately. As he was settling behind his desk, arranging papers, he shared that he had grown up in rural South Carolina, where the lack of enough doctors caused people undue suffering. It had been his desire to be of service to such people. This desire, combined with an interest in science, had led him from South Carolina State College where he majored in Biology with a minor in Chemistry, to Meharry Medical College in Nashville, Tennessee. After receiving his medical degree there, he had done his internship and residency at William Beaumont General Hospital in El Paso, Texas. Following a stint in the service as a physician in Vietnam his last assignment had landed him in Albuquerque, where he decided to remain and set up practice in 1972.

"I sure am glad you did," popped out of my mouth. It was meant most sincerely. I felt a little flustered, since it was my first interview (and a journalist I am not)—but I took a deep breath and dove right in.

"Dr. McIver, I know you are a general surgeon, performing many kinds of surgery, but somewhere along the line you developed a breast care center. I'd like to know more about that, since that's my special interest." The words sounded awkward and pompous to my ears, but he smiled and I felt less nervous.

"Right," he began. "As a general surgeon of course I enjoyed the variety of surgeries and procedures that we were trained to perform, and that we still do perform in the community. But early on, after working with several patients who had the diagnosis of breast cancer, it became of special interest to me. I'm sure that it had to do with the relationships with those earlier patients, and the fact that we did not seem to be making the necessary progress that all would have liked to have seen at that time. I felt that physicians who had a special interest in that area needed to make attempts to concentrate and understand as much as possible about the disease in order to help patients. I just drifted into that direction early in my career, and since that time my practice has evolved to the point where about fifty percent of it is taking care of breast disease."

I was not surprised that so much of his practice was breast care. As far as I am concerned he is the Breast Care King of Albuquerque. I pushed on. "Breast cancer is especially frightening because it seems almost out of control. Statistics at the Tumor Registry at the University of New Mexico Cancer Center indicate breast cancer strikes one in nine women in New Mexico, whereas twenty years ago it was one in twenty." (Now, in 1995, it is one in eight and rising.)

He nodded ruefully. "That's correct."

How terribly frightening are statistics like that! There's a great big mystery there—nobody seems to know why it's increasing so rapidly. Believe it or not, occasionally even men are getting it. But for the moment, I decided to focus on his methods of diagnosis and treatment, getting back to the causes of this problem later.

"Dr. McIver, would you please outline the procedures you follow when someone is referred to you with a breast problem?"

"I think the first and most important step is to establish a good doctor/patient relationship—a rapport with a patient—to understand the patient's concerns and to listen to the patient as well as impart information about the problem. It's very hard to put people at ease in these situations, but one of my objectives is to try to help patients through a very difficult problem—to reduce the stress factor, so to speak, as much as possible."

He paused, regarding me with earnest eyes. "I think that communication is very important—being able to talk with patients and allow them the prerogative to ask questions, to feel free to call up and discuss things, and to try to make them comprehend as much as we presently understand about the problem.

"The patient has to have a chance to enter into making decisions about treatment. That's essential.

"It starts off with the initial examination, of course. And getting to know the patient, the patient's background, history, and other related factors that might be affecting her, or him, at the time. Then it becomes a matter of forming a diagnosis, and there are certain steps and techniques that are fairly routine for doing that part of the evaluation."

I shuddered as I remembered them. "Such as mammograms and biopsies?"

"That's correct. We need to establish a firm, unequivocal diagnosis so that we are sure that the problem we are dealing with is serious—or in a more fortunate situation proving that it is not necessarily serious.

"Once we've established the diagnosis I think it is necessary for the physician to outline the patient's options of therapy and what is being recommended. We need to tell them that we don't have a complete answer now, but we have a combination of therapies that are used in order to control this problem, put it into remission and to cure it. So the approach would be stepwise: getting to know the patient, establishing the diagnosis, and then discussing options of therapy."

I was impressed that he used the Big "C" word. Cure. Not many physicians use that word when they talk about cancer.

"In your particular case, Dr. McIver, surgery is the option, right?"

"Well yes it is, if you look at the history of the management of breast malignancies.

"Other forms of mastectomy had been done before Dr. Halsted, who developed and performed the radical mastectomy nearly a century ago. From then on it was a problem that surgeons dealt with almost exclusively. But now with the advent of drugs and chemotherapy, and a refinement of radiation therapy, there is a team approach to breast cancer treatment. Many times all three of these modalities are combined in order to get a result. And yet the surgeon should remain the captain of the team, so to speak, and the captain of the ship in directing the patient's course—certainly through the early stages of treatment—and coordinating the course of therapy between the radiotherapist, the chemotherapist and the surgical procedure.

"Of course, the initial diagnosis is almost always dependent on a surgical procedure, a basic biopsy of some sort."

Yes, of course. I could not think of any other way to determine for sure whether a breast lump is malignant. "OK, so biopsy and surgery are virtually always the first step?"

"Yes. We are hoping to get to the point where we use a needle biopsy technique, which technically is not surgery, but is still an interventional approach. It is possible that in the future the needle biopsy could even obviate the need for surgical procedures; but that would imply that we have a good modality in the realm of chemotherapy and X-ray that would obliterate the tumors. It still remains a surgical procedure to remove the primary tumor or the tissue that might contain tumor."

The telephone rang, interrupting our conversation. Dr. McIver apologized for the intrusion, but I took advantage of the pause to figure out what to ask him next. He replaced the phone.

"I know there is a choice now in the type of surgical procedure once you have diagnosed a malignancy—whether it is to be a radical mastectomy, modified radical mastectomy or a lumpectomy. What do you think are the results of these different approaches?"

Dr. McIver passed his hands across his curly gray hair, leaning thoughtfully back in his chair. "The National Breast Adjuvant Project, which was instituted back in the 1970s, monitored the method in which patients were treated. They looked at large numbers of patients. I feel one must qualify their results with the fact that all tumors are not the same nor at the same stage when diagnosed; however they found that, stage for stage, more conservative procedures are just as good. In early stage tumors, if the entire tumor is excised it does not imply that the entire breast must be removed. In certain types of tumors and certain stages it has been shown that if you match those people who have been treated with the more radical procedures (such as the old standard radical mastectomy which is the model by which we compared subsequent procedures) the outcome of the lesser procedures such as the modified radical mastectomy is just as good. The radical mastectomy, which is not done much anymore, takes the entire breast, lymph glands and the underlying muscle. The modified radical mastectomy takes the entire breast and nearby lymph glands, but spares the underlying muscle. The lumpectomy removes only the tumor and nearby lymph glands."

I remembered an older friend who had a radical mastectomy over twenty-five years ago. She had described to me the immense difficulty of regaining the use of her arm, as the muscles that control much of the arm's strength and motion had been removed. A fleeting feeling of gratitude warmed me as I became aware of my own, still useful, right arm which was at that moment dutifully involved in taking notes. It helped my hand scribble a series of exclamation points and doodle a few loops and circles. As good as ever before.

Dr. McIver continued, unaware of my mental digression. "Early on in this newer conservative approach it was felt that there were limits as to the size of the tumor that should be treated by lumpectomy. That basic principle still holds to some degree. It gives us the prerogative in certain instances to recommend a lesser procedure if it's a very small tumor. There are several factors to consider, which means that every patient is an individual, and we do individualize the primary treatment when we recommend the most favorable form of therapy. The first criteria that came out was that two centimeters was the upper limit for which we felt a lumpectomy would be appropriate. In recent times, and with the improvement of x-ray therapy, we've extended that and larger tumors can be treated that way."

"If you did a lumpectomy and subsequently the pathology report showed that it was a real aggressive tumor, would you do a second surgery?"

"That's still a controversial point. It depends on the analysis of the tissue. If the malignancy extends to the margins in every aspect of the breast tissue removed, I think most physicians would opt to go back and remove more or all breast tissue.

"I think the principle that we should remember is that the purpose of conservative surgery is to leave a cosmetic result that is acceptable to the patient. All forms of therapy try to accomplish the same medical outcome—surgery by removing all the tumor cells; lumpectomy by removing the major nest of cells and sterilizing the rest of the breast in case there are other tumor cells remaining there. Both forms of therapy try to preserve breast tissue that is free of cancer cells. If too much tissue must be removed to get around a tumor, it will not be cosmetically acceptable, and that would be an unsound choice of therapy. The cosmetic effect could be worse than removing the whole breast."

Intellectually, I understand that we are more than our body parts. I still feel like me, still feel womanly, but I am acutely aware of my lifelong struggle with body image.

Does it begin in infancy with a birth mark or a casual remark about a smelly diaper? Does daddy's "Phew, I'm not touching that!" translate on a felt level into, "What's wrong with me that he doesn't want to touch me?" Self image has murky, unclear origins. For me, having a hysterectomy years earlier had not been a problem, because you can't see that something is missing. Just a faint scar like a wide smile below my stretch marks. But having a breast amputated is entirely different. It's pretty hard to believe you are just as desirable, even to the most loving husband, as you were before. Even when my perfect gentleman of a husband said his only problem with it was where to put his other hand, I still couldn't quite believe him.

I stirred uneasily, adjusting my rear in that soft, brown chair. "Dr. McIver, you are working in an area that is fraught with psychological overtones, emotional overtones. It is involved with the female psyche and our cultural expectations of ourselves—not the same as operating on an arm or a leg. I know that you do surgery compassionately, with the intent of preserving as much of the breast as possible. Or in the case of total mastectomy, facilitating reconstruction and return to normalcy."

"Correct. All those aspects are there. Obviously we would hope that if a person has to have a problem of this nature it can be treated with conservative surgery. Secondly, we want to preserve function. That is part of why we changed over from the old radical mastectomy, which used to debilitate patients quite a bit. Muscles were removed, and we used to try to remove every lymph node in the axilla, which would leave the patient with a lot of arm swelling. We try to perform surgery that will enable cosmetic reconstruction to be done with reasonable results. But we don't want to compromise good therapy in favor of cosmesis. We feel that a patient has either to be cured or placed in remission before cosmetic outcome is considered."

That wonderful "C" word again. I love this man! I pressed on. "How do you decide how many lymph nodes to remove?"

"We usually decide on a certain amount of lymphatic tissue to remove. Lymph nodes vary. They are not a constant number. They are not the same in every individual. In thinking back I believe the largest number of lymph nodes we have ever removed is sixty, and the smallest number is sometimes down to two or three. The technique is that we have to have adequate lymph tissue to evaluate and complete the staging of the patient. That means we stake out a region, so to speak, and remove all the lymph tissue that's in that region. We remove what we call the level one and level two nodes, which are closest to the site, and we leave the level three nodes, which are the highest, farthest away. Based on large studies we feel that if those nodes are negative, there should not be any positive nodes in the more distant level three. Of course in medicine there is nothing one hundred percent. The true reason for removing lymph nodes is to determine the stage of disease in the patient."

My daughter Melanie is a registered nurse. She felt that in order to fight my cancer, I should know as much as possible, so she sent me volumes of medical information that was available to her. According to my loose translation into lay terms, stage one means a simple tumor, with no lymph nodes infected by cancer cells. Stage two means a few lymph nodes are infected. Stage three means many lymph nodes are infected and a there is a possibility the disease is systemic. Stage four means the cancer has spread to other parts of the body.

"The staging, then, would have a great deal to do with deciding what kind of follow-up therapy the patient should undergo?"

"Correct," he affirmed.

"The surgery itself, from my own experience, was not particularly debilitating. It was something I was able to recover from quite quickly."

Dr. McIver smiled. "That's been our experience with most patients. We go into the surgery with the objective that we want to return the patient as close to normal as we can in terms of function, getting around, performing duties and so forth. We realize that with every patient there will be some minimal disability; but the fact that we don't remove the pectoralis major and pectoralis minor muscles and all the nodes means that we do have that option of taking patients through the procedure without debilitating them."

I figured that pretty much covered diagnosis and surgical procedures, so I moved into the area of personal opinion.

"Now getting into the causes, what do you think is the reason that the breast cancer rate has risen so dramatically?"

It was not a question to be answered easily, so his reply was measured and lengthy. "From your reading and exposure too, I'm sure you are aware that this is one of the areas of great concern at the moment—and also an area of great speculation. We have broached the subject several times at different meetings. Our tumor registry, which happens to be an outstanding tumor registry, is looking into the epidemiology and demographics of this to decide which factors are important in this increased incidence. We do believe that it is a true increased incidence. By that I mean it's beyond the fact that we are finding tumors earlier and more frequently with the widespread use of mammography. We do believe that there is an actual, true increase in the numbers of people who are developing tumors. It's not just a reflection of more diagnoses.

"There are several areas that one has to think about. Researchers are looking at things that might be common to large groups, such as dietary problems, certain food intakes. We also have to keep in mind that we are exposed to more chemicals now in many different areas, the environment, even our food products. We are forced to eat a lot of preserved foods, as you know. Yet it may be very difficult to use the epidemiologic studies to pin this down, because it's difficult to know what a person is consuming at a given time and compare that to large numbers of people to determine patterns and habits. So if it is something to do with diet, that may be hard to establish. There are some scientists who feel this may be the source of some of the problem.

"The other part of the question researchers are looking at is, could there be an environmental cause? Perhaps something that we have no control over but are constantly exposed to through our environment—just by being where we are. There may be much in our environment that we know nothing about.

"Another question is, could there be a hormonal relationship? The use of hormones over the years has changed, at least in terms of artificial supplements that we've used. All of these factors are being researched.

"We've gone a long time on the theory that there were viral particles at the basis of tumor formation. We know that we're encountering new kinds of viruses with the AIDS crisis. I think the real question is whether there is some yet undiscovered virus or virus particle that we just haven't been able, through our scientific endeavors, to put our finger on. The conferences I have attended on this have raised more questions than answers. But to get to the bottom of the problem you have first to raise the questions."

The phone rang again, giving me an opportunity to consider his words. When he was finished, he brought his focus back to the room and our conversation. "Where were we?"

I tried to pick up the thread. "Whatever the cause of cancer, as I understand it, there is a change in the cell metabolism. Is that correct?"

"Correct."

"Something produces that change," I continued. "Could it be a genetic kind of thing? A gene pattern?"

"That is the basis of another area of research. They are trying to do gene studies of all of mankind, to try to map out every gene a person has. They are looking for where this starts, whether there is some outside mechanism that triggers a defective gene or cell. There is certain research work now that strongly supports the fact that some cancer patients have a certain gene pattern. There may be a defect that is passed along on a hereditary basis that, if the right set of circumstances occurs, or if the right milieu should occur, a group of cells in a particular individual will undergo uncontrolled change and develop into cancer. So there may be some genetic basis that might be a factor, which again we haven't sorted out carefully enough." (Since this conversation, scientists have announced the discovery of a gene that predisposes to breast cancer.)

I thought of my mother, alive and well in her nineties. My grandmother and grandfather too, who both lived into their nineties. My family tree should be the Sequoia. Where was a genetic weakness? All I could think of in my case that might have caused this problem was radiation therapy for acne as a teenager and a bout of mastitis while nursing my daughter Alissa. I wondered aloud, "Aren't there other things that alter genes too, like radiation?"

He nodded. "Correct, which may again bring in the environment. That may be the mechanism by which this occurs: chemicals or other things in the environment that we come in contact with may damage the genes, resulting in uncontrolled growth. Uncontrolled growth is what cancer is all about."

"Now for the really big question, Dr. McIver. What do you think will be the cure for cancer? How do you think it will come? Through gene therapy that they are getting excited about now, or anti-viral research, perhaps?"

"Anti-viral—working with the immune system—looking at the genetic pattern—of course, all this ties in. One would hope that we could find the defective gene, if that is the problem, and be able to have a test that would point this out. But it would have to parallel something that we could do immediately to treat the problem, to block development of the particular tumor. You would hope that it would be something that could be done on a very simple level, a simple medication."

"Or a simple food, like eating lots of broccoli." Wishful thinking on my part. He laughed politely at my joking.

Pressing on, I asked him about something of special interest to me. "Dr. McIver, do you see a connection between mental attitude and disease, as either a cause or affecting the outcome?"

"In my medical school training," he replied, "we had what was called an integrated curriculum, where we studied mental attitudes in emotional stress and disease, along with our basic learning about medicine. That kind of impressed me about our curriculum. We had four years of integrated psychiatry, which meant that we looked at the emotional side of problems. I'm a firm believer that there is a connection between the stress mechanism and the body. By that I mean what we are thinking and doing in the situations that confront us on a day-to-day basis, and the way we deal with problems and diseases. I do think there is a connection, and I think it's important that both of these aspects, the physical and the emotional, be addressed when the patient is being treated. That's why we feel that imparting as much information as you can to the patient is important, because the mind does begin to play tricks on you. You imagine all sorts of things. We have to admit to patients that although we do not have all of the answers, don't understand all the processes, yet we have studied this long enough to have some ideas and concepts that we think will help them deal with their problem. We give them information, rather than let their imagination run away with them. That's an important part of the treatment, to deal with the stress that is created from the illness."

"Bottom line, Dr. McIver, are the survival rates for breast cancer increasing?"

"We would like to believe that, but we don't yet have large groups of statistics. I can't help but believe that the intervention of the mammogram and the more up-front attitude about this problem that patients have must improve the survival rate and the cure rate. I can't quote you a study right now, because all these are in process. As far as breast tumors are concerned, you have to look at the fifteen-year studies and the twenty-year studies to be absolutely sure. We do have studies now that have been going on for about twelve years. Although we have seen more diagnoses, we think that a larger number of these patients that are being diagnosed early will be cured, and will be in that improved survival rate that you are asking about.

"Certainly it is bound to change, although you hear a lot of pessimistic reporting saying this hasn't changed significantly. I think that is a time-related thing. I think that in the next few years you are going to see that large numbers of patients are doing well."

I hate statistics with a passion. You can make them prove anything you want them to prove; and since they are based on past information they are never reflective of what's happening at the present, right now. "Obviously, there is a time lag between the statistics and being able to make any sense out of them," I said.

"That's true."

Many women among my friends and acquaintances have had breast cancer. A lot of them are artists, although I'm not sure the cancer has anything to do with their profession. Some of them are sick and living with cancer, but the majority of them are disease-free and doing well. Perhaps I'm an optimist, but I ventured my opinion in hopes Dr. McIver would concur:

"I would like to believe that the improvement of techniques to treat breast cancer will help to increase the survival rate. I have heard a lot of negative reports, yet somehow it does feel like there's a lot more hope than there used to be. This is from my observation of the many people I know who have had breast cancer."

He didn't disappoint me. "We think so. We can't certainly say that everything we're doing hasn't changed anything from the early 1960s. I have to feel, I have to believe, that patients are doing much better with this problem than they were in those days. I must admit that a lot of those patients waited longer to come in, because of the attitude about breast cancer at that time. Since this has changed for the better, people are coming in much earlier. That has to make an impact on the survival rate."

"What advice would you give to women about how to avoid breast cancer? What message would you like them to hear?"

Dr. McIver considered his answer. "I think it's important to keep up with the latest opinions that are coming to us out of research," he said at length. "Valuable information comes out of tumor registries and things of that sort. The information that comes out of the newspapers and medical writers who write a story just to make a deadline for a fee is much less valuable.

"I think the message that would come out of this would have to be to change those things that we can change based on our lifestyle. We don't like to get on a soap box about certain lifestyles that we know are detrimental to people's health. Everybody knows about smoking and high fat diets and all those things we think in an indirect way may damage our genes.

"So I think women need to look at those reports and evaluate whether they are reports from valid sources that have a true interest in the problem and have really researched it. I suggest that they should try to stay away from the sensational, like the magazines where writers are not necessarily interested in the outcome of people's health—they are interested in the income from their article, or whatever. People have to scrutinize all the material they are confronted with and say "Is this believable? Does this sound real or possible?" And try to respect some of the recommendations that are made. I think that women should keep up with reading about future approaches to the problem, the use of tamoxifen, for example, and see if good basic research is being done.

"If people are in a group at high risk, based on family history or findings at examination or changes in the mammograms, they really need to maintain good follow-up, stay with the problem and avoid those things that we think might be contributing to the development of breast cancer. That's important."

"So you are saying, really, that women need to take responsibility for informing themselves and seeing through the screen of disinformation."

"That is correct, and they must decide which routes they are going to follow with this problem, because there are a lot of people imparting information based on knowledge of just one case—based on the exposure to one relative or one friend. I don't know why some people find a need to tell the worst story they have heard. They don't always come up to you and say, 'Well, my friend had this problem and she's doing great—she has been doing great for years.' They would much rather come up and tell you horror stories, and I have never understood that."

It was all too easy to call to mind the cancer dirges I had heard when I was most vulnerable. "One of the things that I found out is that you don't have much in the way of emotional barriers when you are in that situation. You can respond very positively to people who are bringing good information, but also it can wipe you out if people bring you their tales of disaster. I learned that real fast. And painfully.

"But back to your advice, Dr. McIver: whatever is generally good for your health, taking care of your nutrition, adequate rest, trying to resolve the stresses in your life, keeping your liver in good detoxifying form—"

"Good lifestyle," he added, "good living—and of course that means different things to different people. Keeping up with literature on new research, always with an awareness of the source. You certainly don't read articles from people who are representing the tobacco company to know whether you should smoke or not."

Our scheduled time was running out, but there were a couple of questions I still wanted to ask.

"About mammograms, what do you recommend as a course to follow? When should women begin having mammograms, and how often should they have them?"

"This is a situation that is constantly being reviewed, the way all of our procedures are in medicine—at least all should be. Nothing is set in concrete in terms of recommendations or guidelines. We are seeing a changing pattern with this problem, and there is some thought that the frequency with which we do mammograms might also need to change. For instance, we are seeing a larger number of younger patients with the diagnosis. At the present time doctors are given the prerogative to recommend a mammogram every one to two years between the ages of thirty-five and fifty. After fifty the mammogram really should be done once a year. The incidence of breast cancer seems to be a little higher after fifty, although it is shown that many of these tumors are not as rapidly developing."

I thought of the millions of women who have fibrocystic breast disease. "What about fibrocystic breast disease? Does that have any relationship to breast cancer?"

"Yes it does, but that has to be qualified. There are two kinds of fibrocystic problems. Fortunately, the majority of women have the garden variety type of cystic, tender breasts, swelling in relation to hormones—the tender, lumpy breast syndrome. That does not predispose to breast cancer. That's a hormonal response and reaction.

"But there are patients who have the so-called proliferative fibrocystic pattern. We do think they are at higher risk. Fortunately, they are only about fifteen percent of those who are diagnosed with fibrocystic breast disease. They are at risk, but the only way that could be documented is with a biopsy to determine the pattern. You can draw certain conclusions from a mammogram, but by and large, that type of fibrocystic breast disease has to be diagnosed with a biopsy. If you have the proliferative fibrocystic, yes—that is at a higher risk of developing breast tumors. If it's what we call the garden variety, common type, we're not sure those patients are at increased risk."

"And mastitis? Is there any connection? I had mastitis many years ago in the general area of my tumor."

"There is some concern about inflammation and infection as setting the stage for damaged tissue in that area. But they have not documented that in large studies."

I recalled my own unfortunate experience with the lump that should have been biopsied many months earlier. "Dr. McIver, when do you think a woman should have a lump biopsied?"

"There are certain guidelines that we like to use. There are some lumps that we feel on an examination should be biopsied promptly. There are other kinds of lumps that have certain characteristics, feel a certain way, that are cystic. In those cases a simple aspiration in the office is the best approach to deal with that. If you get fluid out and the lump goes away, then you have resolved the problem.

"Then there are some others which we call indeterminate type lumps that we don't feel are suspicious, but nevertheless they are a lump different from the rest of the architecture of the breast. We feel that kind can be followed over a period of time, but probably the reexamination should not go beyond a two-month period. The same physician should examine again in two months, and if it has not changed or become more discreet, then a biopsy should be done at that point."

"When you do an aspiration in the office, do you biopsy the fluid?"

"We do send the fluid for what we call cell cytology, if it's a first-time biopsy. If it's a patient who has had a chronic fibrocystic problem with many cysts, multiple cysts, then we can in many instances look at the fluid and determine that it doesn't show any cells. That fluid isn't necessarily analyzed. But if it's a first-time cyst or has strange components in it, then it will be analyzed."

"Then this is one form of biopsy?"

"It's a needle biopsy."

"Then the other biopsy would be a surgical excision of the breast lump and a pathology report," I remarked.

"With the breast at all costs we try to excise the whole lump, not just a little portion of the lump. We need to use an excisional technique, then take it apart, identify it and recommend treatment."

From my own experience, I know the fear when you feel a lump; but I think millions of women who have breast lumps may ignore them, not only because they are afraid, but also because they don't know what to do about it. They don't know who to see, or how to go about it. I say to them, it won't get any better if you just worry about it. You have to do something, or you are making a decision to die. Many women really don't know how to find a physician who knows much about breast care. So I asked Dr. McIver, as I folded up my notebook and put away my pen, "Suppose a woman has a breast lump and does not have a doctor to refer her to a surgeon who is knowledgeable in breast care. How would she go about finding such a surgeon to check out her problem?"

"I guess the standard answer for that," he replied, "is to call the Medical Society or the Cancer registry. They know in a surface way which physicians specialize in specific problems. We're not sure that system has been the best in the past. Many of the hospital systems have developed referral patterns, and of course they work more closely with the doctors on the staff of that particular hospital or medical center. They know the special interests and they know the doctors' records of dealing with these kinds of problems. I don't know if this is available all over the country, but in our area there is a physician finder service that each hospital has set up, and we think that probably gets closer to a good referral. The best result may be to call the hospital in your area. They can make a number of recommendations."

"And then to find out for sure," I smiled, "you ask a nurse. That's our grassroots system. They know, because they see the doctors at work, and the results."

Dr. McIver chuckled as he rose to see me to the door. "That's basically correct," he agreed.

I left the interview feeling he had shared a lot of up-to-date information about breast cancer, sweeping away some of the cobwebs. I guess one is more receptive to objective information when feeling healthy. Nearly two years before, while I was going through the diagnosis procedures, a dark veil of fear had colored all my awareness, as I sank into my personal well of despair. Positive information had helped a little, but negative data almost drowned me. Most of the information I received from books about breast cancer focused on statistics. I was not in the hopeful categories. I was in the bad ones. I knew it was time to flounder to the surface or sink under. Some innate drive took over, and the mouse in me became a lion roaring, "I am not a statistic. I am not, not, not a statistic. I am me, damnit!"

It helped. By the time I was ready to see the oncologist, I was determined to get well. I knew that on my journey to recovery, the landscape of fears and hopes still lay before me, hills and valleys to traverse, cliffs to climb, rivers to cross, gradually leading up to that Grand Canyon of Western medicine, chemotherapy.

But lucky for me, the colorful Painted Desert lay just ahead.

Beginning to Understand the Route

D O R O T H E E   L . M E L L A

The Transpersonal Counselor &
Analyst in Color Psychology

I was not housebound for the first week after my mastectomy, but there were two drains attached to the incision, which had to be emptied regularly. Each time, I recorded the amount of lymph they contained—a technique a nurse had taught me in the hospital. Taking the advice of a friend who had recently undergone the same surgery, I put the ends of the drains in a fanny pack around my waist, so they didn't hang down loosely. This solved the flapping-around problem, but sleeping on them was impossible. So I took up residence in a big old velvet recliner in the living room until the drains were removed. Here I slept, watched TV, held court with visitors and provided lap space for a cat and a dog. They should be listed among my healers, for indeed unconditional love is a source of healing. So here's to Missy and Rags, our dogs; and Krutsch and Thunder, our cats—my four-legged healers.

I want to emphasize, for anyone who may need to go through it, that having a mastectomy is not as tough to undergo as more difficult internal operations. One recovers quickly. I spent only one full day after the operation in the hospital. Three days post-mastectomy Toni and I went to get our hair done, and Ted and I went for a walk. Two days later Ted and I hiked out on the mesa—the shrubby high desert wilderness just blocks from our door. That same day he drove me to the grocery store and I did some shopping. The next day I went walking by myself for nearly an hour and I started painting again. I could drive after a week, and although I needed a little more rest than usual, I felt fine and free of pain.

It was during that week after surgery that I became conscious of a process that some might call coincidence, but I call synchronicity. Whatever information you need appears, almost magically, if you are alert to it. This wonderful synchronicity has continued and even escalated to a point that I am now wildly crazy about the marvelous happenings that continue to unfold, more and more often, as I become more aware.

Here is one example. My mother's hairdresser told me about her aunt, whose cancer was kept in remission for years by drinking a tea made from the herb chaparral—until she participated in a research project that required her to go off the tea. She then died within a few weeks. This conversation activated a memory of a book I had read years before, by Ruth Montgomery, called *Threshold to Tomorrow*. In this book, Montgomery tells the story of Jason Winters, who had concocted a tea which dramatically cured him. Doctors had declared his cancer terminal and had given him only weeks to live. This was many years ago, and the now-knighted Sir Jason Winters is still in business. The tea consisted of chaparral, red clover and a special "secret spice" from the Orient. Winters had begun making the tea for others, then marketed it commercially. Would I be able to locate some? Of course. On my next visit to a local health food store I found they had been carrying it for years.

At this writing the FDA has taken ingested chaparral off the market because a few people, I was told, who self-medicated with megadoses, developed liver toxicity. Never mind that thousands, probably hundreds of thousands, of people have used it for many generations without ill effects and with highly beneficial results. This upsets me personally, because on the other hand, the FDA licenses therapeutic use of such life-threatening drugs as adriamycin—and hundreds more—which are administered to thousands of people every day. Certainly, they have therapeutic usefulness, but how many develop toxicity from them?

Anyway, I sat down that very evening to drink my first cup of Jason Winters tea, when a gentleman from Edmonton, Alberta, called about a book that Betty Rice, Norma Milanovich and I had co-authored. The book is called *We, the Arcturians*. This man had opened the book to a page which described himself in perfect detail, and he got excited enough to phone me. In our conversation he mentioned experiments being conducted at the University of Alberta Medical School using magnets to drive medication into the body. For instance, he said, "You can place Jason Winters Tea on the affected area—"

Clang. A door blew open in my head. I nearly choked on my tea. Out came all my troubles, pouring into the ears of this stranger. By the time our conversation ended he had provided me with a long list of resource people and their phone numbers. My follow-up telephone calls produced information on nutrition and alternative cancer therapies that set me on course. At last. Something I could do for *myself*. Right away I began modifying my diet. First to go were fats, sugars and alcohol. Raw food and whole grains became my staples. I quickly slimmed down ten pounds.

Another way to express this wonderful synchronicity is embodied in the old saying, "When the student is ready, the teacher appears." On the day I received my pathology report, needing a teacher, I telephoned Dottee Mella.

I had known Dottee long before I decided to see her for therapy. We both belong to SLMM, the Society of Layerists in Multi Media, which is a National organization of professional artists who work in layers as metaphor. The members are aware of art as an avenue of healing, and the organization forms a network of friendship and support. During my chemotherapy, at a National meeting and symposium on Art and Healing, they formed a prayer circle for me and others needing help. My friend Mary Carroll Nelson, the founder of SLMM, suggested I see Dottee. She felt Dottee would have a special message for me, as Dottee is a breast cancer survivor herself.

Dottee Mella is what one might call a transpersonal counselor, using her knowledge of color psychology, gemstones, and her intuitive abilities, to help people understand their problems and work through them.

Her warm and upbeat manner on the telephone lifted my spirits immediately. She told me to be very positive and not to accept anything without questioning. Question everything. She said that I am to be living proof that illness can only be changed by going inside oneself. I must find the hurt that was probably stuffed away inside and is surfacing now as illness. I must identify it, embrace it, understand it, express it—feel the sorrow, the anger; bring it forward to the now time and forgive myself and the world.

"Hold it, Dottee," I blurted into the phone. Her words had evoked a sudden flash of memory, something I had indeed swallowed and forgotten. Right then and there I was ten years old again and an old sea captain I met on a deserted path in Canada was grabbing my growing breasts and holding me captive for what seemed an eternity. He kept saying, "Now aren't you getting to be a fine, big, American girl."

Shame—terror—powerlessness—violation. I wanted to *die.* When he finally let me go, I ran home in tears. I couldn't tell anyone—especially my parents. We didn't talk about such things. I was terrified. I felt defiled, and horribly guilty, as if somehow my budding awareness of sexuality had provoked the attack. I remembered hiding in my room thinking this awful, dirty thing showed all over me. I was truly devastated.

Remembering this incident on the phone with Dottee brought back a rush of emotions, as real as if it were happening all over again. In a flash I relived the dread as he approached me, the fear knotting my stomach, his sinister leering smile, his big callused hands. I even recalled his smell, musty, evil; and my terror as he held me prisoner.

But now, as an adult, I felt intense anger instead of shame. *That dirty old man. Where did he get off doing that to a little girl?*

Later on in life other men had grabbed and held me: the father of one of my teenage friends, my own uncle, the man who lived next door. In college I was raped on a date. Each time I was powerless, unable to defend myself. Each time I was ashamed. All I could do was get away as fast as I could and never say anything to anyone about what had happened. I "swallowed" it. I forgot it. And now I was wondering if—in a different way—it was attacking me all over again.

I put down the telephone with a sense of wonderment, anticipating Dottee's promised visit to my home.

Six days after surgery, the same day that I had my first appointment with the medical oncologist, Dottee came to my house to work with me. Dr. Saiki had given me an awareness of what I was in for during chemotherapy, and it was pretty grim. But that afternoon, Dottee and I sat in the sunshine of my studio and she painted another, brighter picture. According to Dottee, I could heal myself by balancing what has been out of balance: my feelings of powerlessness and lack of self love.

If you can imagine a "colorful" person, that's Dottee. She radiates warmth, vitality and light, from the colorful clothes she wears to her short, bright blond hair and sparkling eyes. We went right to work. I was handed a box of crayons and several pages of blank circles. "What color do you think of when you feel hungry?" I was to fill in a circle with that color. "What color do you think of when you think of coolness?" Fill in another circle. And so on for two pages of circles. This is what she calls her SICA, or color self-portrait, which she uses along with her intuitive perception to determine what emotional areas need balancing with external circumstances. If you think this is easy, kindergarten stuff, think again. As an artist, I work with color all the time, but I was hard put to express my thoughts and feelings with appropriate Crayola.

After the SICA analysis, Dottee informed me I ought to wear pink, for self-nurturing. I should carry the gemstones she gave me for peace, inspiration and healing, and I should repeat a special affirmation every day.

Dottee told me her own breast cancer experience. She had been healed by surgery and radiation therapy, nutritional support, plus lots of personal work to bring herself into balance and get rid of hidden, destructive emotions. Amazing to me was how she guided me to envision some of my "past lives." She visualized me as an Egyptian priest/healer, an English author/playwright, an artist, and an ancient Atlantean scientist. Well, I didn't remember any of these lives, but I do have a great interest in Egyptian antiquities. I also have dabbled in writing all my life, I am an artist, and I have always been fascinated by the mysteries of lost civilizations—hmm.

Her visit left me riding a wave of hope, and savoring her parting words: "You are going to emerge victorious and become a healer yourself."

I saw Dottee professionally more than a half dozen times over the next year. During each session she first informed me as to what was happening in the Cosmos and in our lives. "As above, so below." Each session contained another SICA, to see what progress I was making in harmonizing my inner emotions with my outward life.

On top of that I was given good advice about dealing with the events and people in my environment. She told me colors to wear (primarily pink, peach or rose for self-nurturing and green for healing). Before I started radiation, Dottee prepared me by citing her own experiences and the things she did to cleanse herself of the toxins that are its by-product. She gave me special gemstones to keep my personal electromagnetic field in order, because according to her, radiation blows it out of whack. Each session left me feeling optimistic and empowered, and I really needed that. I learned positive thinking is a vital part of healing, because if you don't think you can be healed, you won't be healed.

Dottee suggested I visualize the cancer cells being destroyed by light and washed from my body, so I developed a ritual that was performed (at first hesitantly; then later, with more confidence) in the shower. Native American spirituality has long attracted me, so my ritual consisted of facing each of the directions and chanting a Cherokee song of respect. The words or notes really don't matter (or the singing voice)—it's probably the intention that counts.

Then I call upon the power of each direction. East is the power of being in the moment, light streaming in. South signifies trust, rest and refreshment. West is death and rebirth, transformation. North is guidance and direction. Father Sky is seminal energy, and Mother Earth is manifesting energy. I call upon the power of these six sacred directions, and bring them through me, for I am (we all are) the seventh sacred direction. By that I mean we are all connected to the natural forces of our environment and therefore part of them.

In that moment of power, I speak affirmations about being healed and visualize my body filled with bubbling emerald green light. I inhale sparkling golden light and as I exhale I imagine the golden light pressing that green light (with all the cancer cells, toxins and dead cells incorporated into it) down through my body, out through my toes, and down the drain.

Then, since nature abhors a vacuum, I breathe in that sparkling golden light and fill my body with it, nourishing all the "little flowers" of healthy new cells. I emerge from the shower clean, balanced and renewed. This meditation could be performed anywhere at all. But for me, it just feels right to do it in the cleansing, purifying warm water of my daily shower.

CONVERSATION WITH DOROTHEE MELLA

When I walked into Dottee's office for our interview, she greeted me with her usual big hug. I had already navigated through the menagerie of animals surrounding her home and office—horses, ducks, dogs—all as much a part of Dottee as her colors, candles and gems. Ramona, Dottee's secretary, brought us some coffee—decaf but strong and warming. A computer on which Dottee's numerous books take form inhabits the office, along with rocks and crystals of every description. Mementos, souvenirs, newspaper clippings and photographs plaster the walls. The net effect is rather like being inside a glass sculpture, intimate yet expansive. This habitat is where she counsels clients, helping them see the underlying causes of their distress and giving them tools to destroy the roots.

Dottee closed the door, lit the candle on a small round table, put a tape in her recorder, leaned forward with her hands clasped on the table, raised her eyebrows and said, "Well?"

I laughed. "Well—you already told me that your job here was to help others see clearly, and I really think that's wonderful, because that is certainly what you did for me. How do you do it?"

"I use the tools of the arts. The artist sees. What is within is without. What is outside is within."

After being with Dottee so many times, I knew what she meant, but I thought it could still use some clarification. "Would you explain how it works, for people who haven't any background in this?"

"Yes. Many years ago I devised with art students a method of formulating a language of color, not knowing exactly at that time its application or usage. I gathered tons of material about what people identified with when they thought about certain colors. If they were sleepy, what color would they identify with?—and on and on. Suddenly it occurred to me that with certain colors people would use the words 'I think' and with other colors they would say 'I feel' and they were coming from different parts of a person. They were coming from the mind (I think) and they were coming from the human response system (I feel). So I put a manual together that became a self portrait technique, based on 'I think I am—' and 'I feel I am—.'

"By putting together external circumstances with the thoughts and feelings expressed in response to colors, you could see if the external and the internal were synchronized and in harmony with each other, or were different faces of the Adam or Eve. If they were different, you could help them see clearly by showing them what was really going on within themselves. So that's how it worked—it was a self portrait.

"Because society demanded that you didn't get into the human response system with an individual unless they go through therapy, I created it as a color analysis. People could take the responsibility to see themselves clearly and feel good about themselves, wearing the right colors. For example, if someone had a vivid imagination but never realized it, how wonderful that the color analysis said, 'Look, you have a vivid imagination. You are very creative. So why don't you use this talent in everyday life?' It would motivate a person to help himself or herself."

I was aware this was a different color analysis from what people are used to, where they pull out color swatches when they go shopping and use words like "summer, winter, spring and fall." This color analysis was more in the realm of psychology, but I knew it went past that. I started to summarize her words: "So your response to their choices helped them to understand things about themselves they were not aware of—"

"Yes. Their response to their color choices helped them to see themselves. I put the system on computer in 1979 so that other people could analyze the SICA. But I have an intuitive gift of insight, so I could go deeper. If a person was not responding to himself or herself I could rip the veil off and say, 'Hey! Take a real good look at what you are creating from within yourself. And by the time it gets out here, you are going to have to face it.' "

I well remembered. "You ripped off a veil for me just merely talking on the telephone. I don't know how you did that, but I flashed on an incident that occurred to me long ago. Now I understand how it has affected me, but it was forgotten until that moment."

"Exactly. What I do with clients is stimulate them like an art teacher would stimulate a student. I could help paint their painting, but a good art teacher never puts her hands on other people's work. She can demonstrate how to put a dewdrop on a rose, but she should not do it for them."

I put my coffee cup down on the table, tapping a punctuation mark onto the tape recording. "So what you are saying is you can give people insight, but they have to do the work themselves."

"Yes. They must take the responsibility. They are not my children, nor my students. They come to me for a one-shot deal, to peel back the banana and take a look. I will be there, I will support them until they are able to peel the whole banana back themselves."

I was interested in how her research leading to the SICA came into being. I knew it was long before color analysis was fashionable, so what prompted her awareness at that time? I pressed her for more details.

Dottee took off her glasses and closed her eyes as if she were projecting herself back in time. "Well, it came to me through a spiritual experience. It was when I was teaching at an art school. I was given the responsibility of planning all the classes for teachers and curriculum for students; therefore I only taught three classes a week. Because my teaching load was minimal all the difficult students were put into my classes.

"I had awful students. Not really awful, because they turned out to be magnificent students. But they certainly were a mixed bag of humanity. I couldn't get through to any of them. They were running out at lunch and shooting themselves up with drugs, or the retired colonels were coming in, either patronizing me or philosophizing in class how awful the hippie generation was. It was really bad news. I was pretty depressed.

"I was directed by an inner voice. One particularly frustrating day I came home from class and threw myself across the bed in despair. I heard a voice telling me to get up and go to the library, a certain library, in another district far away. I was to find a specific book, the only book of its kind translated from French.

"It was pretty dramatic. I realized at the time that it was Divine guidance. I knew that if I didn't follow this direction I would be going the wrong way. It was against my husband's advice. Who could blame him? He really thought I was nuts, hearing a voice and getting orders from—who?—what?" She opened her eyes, bright with laughter.

What an experience, I thought. "What was the book?"

"It was the spiritual writings or journals of the great artist, Vasily Kandinsky. I've never been able to find the book since; it disappeared a year later from the library.

"I did not realize until ten years ago that he was one of the first originators of the language of color. It just blew my mind. But this happened way back, twenty-some years ago.

"Anyway, I was only allowed to take the book out for two weeks. I didn't know what this book was supposed to do for me. I thought that maybe through osmosis I'd absorb something from it, so I just toted it around everywhere with me. I even slept on it. I had no idea of what I was looking for. And nothing special happened. But the last day before I had to take it back, while I was having a cup of coffee, the book opened five times. On its own.

"At least, I saw the book open on its own. At that time I was in the habit of opening a Bible or a book I was reading every day and getting a message from a line on that page. That was how I got my daily inspiration. So it wasn't unusual for me to look for messages in this book that was opening for me.

"Here were my messages, five of them. However, I couldn't interpret them. All I could do was copy them from the book. They were in bold, powerful, magnified print while the rest of the page was blurry. I could read them, but I couldn't understand them. So I wrote down these five messages in a little notebook—I still have the notebook—and then took the book back to the library, still not knowing what I was supposed to get from this.

"On the way home I decided to stop for a haircut. Because it was a wintry day and my hair was still damp, I was sitting under an old-fashioned hair dryer before going back outside. I thought about the little notebook I had written those five sentences in, so I pulled it out of my purse. The first sentence was:

'Color has a mysterious power. It is the key, touched by man, to open him to his soul.'

"Suddenly the message was clear. I thought *My God, how simple. How simple.* Then the next sentence was:

'An artist sees what will be and makes it seen to the world.'

"My skin was prickling all over. The next day I went to school and said to these students, 'I'm not going to really teach you technique. What I'm going to do is let you learn to express yourself.

" 'I want you to take a walk in the woods with me and pick one color for your woods. Describe your woods by telling me just one color. Are your woods green, or white in the winter? Or whatever. Then make a brand new palette. Make four colors that are contrasting and four colors that will harmonize with it and put all these colors on a canvas.'

"They were too busy to fight or anything. Our routine was that in the last half hour of class, all the paintings were lined up and we all became judge and jury. Everybody began to talk at once and the colonel said to the hippie 'My God, you've been in my woods. Your painting looks exactly like mine.' Then they all started communicating with each other.

"I tried it with all of my three classes. They just opened up. The dean called me down and asked me what I was doing. I said I didn't know. He accused me of practicing astrology in my classes."

I realized it was a long time ago, and now people have a much more enlightened attitude about things that can't be felt or seen; but to confuse astrology and psychology—and to find the emotions of color offensive in an art school? Art is supposed to be on the leading edge of culture.

"So anyway," Dottee continued, "this started me on the career of color, and I just started peeling the banana back. The SICA came into being about two years later. SICA stands for Self Image Color Analysis. We call it the self portrait technique because people don't come for a color analysis, which is finding out what colors suit their complexion, etc. I chose to use color as therapy to help people see clearly.

"First of all, you give people insight. Then you stimulate their creativity to help themselves. And then you make it enjoyable. You make it fun. That's the art of living. We do the self portrait so people can understand themselves—'Mirror, mirror on the wall—I'm a wonderful communicator but I'm not using my ability to communicate.' Then we use color as a practical aid. That means colors in the wardrobe should be used with purpose, functionally. Colors in the environment should also be used with purpose. Then we use the mind to create, with focusing tools such as colored candles and positive affirmations. That's why I wrote my books on Candle Power."

I wanted specific information as to how this color thing worked. "When you talk about the practical uses of color, how does that work? On a mental level? On a physical level?"

Dottee shook her head. "No, it works on a human response level. Color is light, reflected and refracted. That means as the sun's ray comes into our atmosphere it is bent, and that bent light is absorbed into different materials. So when we see color we are seeing the ray of the sun that is not absorbed.

"In other words, when we are seeing a pink blouse, the color pink is reflected to our eyes, and the rest of the rainbow is being absorbed by the fabric. Light enters the eye, hits the 'movie screen,' then bounces through the optic nerve to the brain. It is the brain that sees color. The eye doesn't really see color, it permits the light to enter.

"What we see is often what we need," she pursued, "so the SICA will give us practical information on what colors to wear on the body because we are in need of those colors. As an example, people who are very sensitive, very emotional, need to wear darker shades of color because it blocks out interfering energy coming from the outside. In that particular case color acts as a barrier.

"Compare color to a skin creme. Some people's skin absorbs more of the moisturizer than others. Some people do not need certain skin cremes, but need others.

"Color is absorbed into the body. The brain sees color, but the skin also absorbs color. The colors that you place on the body are absorbed as fractures of light into the energy system of the body, according to what you would need."

Wow. This was a new concept for me. I started to get excited. "In other words, the skin takes from the colors what the body needs?"

Dottee took a sip of coffee and replaced her mug with authority. "Exactly. A very sensitive person needs darker colors. A very strong, powerful person may need some lighter colors. A person who is despondent and depressed may need some 'up' colors. A person who is too excited may need some 'down' colors. The colors can be used as a 'skin creme' for balance."

I am still trying to figure this out. The "little professor" inside my head is fascinated. "I'm trying to understand if this works on an emotional basis, a physical basis—"

"A human response basis," she interrupted, eager to make this clear to me. "What is human response? What is the mind? Tell me what the mind is."

"I would say the controlling intellect—"

"And it houses the soul. So you have higher mind which houses the soul, and then the intellect, which is housed within the brain. The intellect has the capability of interpreting, analyzing, communicating, building, forming. Forming, forming, forming. Mind."

Her voice rose in intensity. "Mind doesn't feel, the human response system does. Human response is a system of energy fed by the five senses that responds to outside energies and to energies from within the self. It's this response that creates emotions.

"If I pinch you, what are you going to do? Say ouch and get irritated? Your internal reaction is emotional. If I say 'I love you,' what are you going to do? Your reaction will also be emotional, but different.

"Your human response system recognizes whether it's an 'ouch' or an 'I love you.' Both emotions have an effect upon the body."

I remembered the many "ouches" I had received, and how I had believed it was okay because I could handle them—rise above them as church and culture said we should. Turn the other cheek. Be noble. Be good. Be strong. Endure. Be holy. Let yourself be hurt rather than hurt anyone else's feelings. Above all, don't hurt anyone's feelings. Be a peacemaker. I groaned inwardly. Were all those "right" things wrong? Only if they weren't my true feelings, according to Dottee.

As the afternoon sunlight began to warm the table where we were sitting, light was entering my brain and peeling away yet another layer. It felt good. It felt a little less dense.

"The mind has an effect on the human response system," Dottee continued. "If we are pinched all the time the human response system gets used to accepting the pinch. Ouch. Ouch. Ouch. Ouch. Ouch. We begin to feel that 'nobody loves me' or 'life gives me pain.' It hurts the body because the body says 'Oh my God I'm in pain all the time.' But the mind doesn't know it.

"That's why we have to change the attitude. The SICA changes attitudes just by helping people to understand what they really feel. Next, the SICA indicates what colors to wear to help change those ouchies; and then we give you tools to focus the mind towards changing the attitude."

I intuitively felt that the ouches and our response to them underlie disease. Dis-ease. "I think we are close here to the connection with cancer—"

"Yes."

"—and I would like your thoughts on how it develops."

Speaking in measured tones, Dottee began to explain. "In the human response system, the division between 'I think I am' and 'I feel I am' creates a division within the body in the cellular structure.

"In other words, if the mind is saying 'I can do it, there's no ouches' —and the feelings are saying 'Ouch! Ouch! Ouch!'—it sends signals to the body. I'm no scientist, so I can't tell you if it's through the peripheral nervous system, the central nervous system, autonomic nervous system or whatever—but it's like misfiring.

"It creates a constant misfiring, and this constant misfiring between what you think and what you feel begins to break down the energy balance within a cell. One cell begins to break down and then a whole bunch of cells begin to break down and pretty soon you have an illness.

"Incidents in our lives when we feel a loss and say 'It's OK,' or hurt ourselves rather than hurt others, also contribute to disease. It takes years. It may take twenty years or more for a tumor or an illness to develop. And the only way to remove the causal root is to see clearly. We can't band-aid cancer. We can't cover it up and say it doesn't exist. I'm not talking about denial of the disease—I'm talking about denial of the person. We create it in the breast, we create it in the brain—"

"So you're saying that no therapy will cure it unless—"

"—people get in touch with themselves."

"And getting in touch with yourself restores balance?"

"Yes. You start life with it. You had it."

I shook my head. "I lost it somewhere."

"Because you put yourself in a position of servitude, when inside yourself you knew you were not. Once you became the creator as an artist you opened, and you could no longer have that division within yourself. You had to pull it together. You had to acknowledge it. Once it's acknowledged—"

"Then healing can progress?"

She leaned forward, looking at me intently, brown eyes flashing. "Of course. Because we change the energy. Instead of short circuiting, it's flowing.

"Unless you can see why the cancer came you cannot heal it. You have to look inside. There has to be no division. Divinity is in everything, so it is within ourselves as well as outside ourselves. If we can put the Divinity within ourselves together with the Divinity outside ourselves, we are healing the division.

"The moment we say 'Please, help me,' we are sticking God right back outside ourselves. The true attitude is to recognize that we are the creators."

I knew this was true, but a heavy responsibility. "A lot of people don't want to accept that because they feel guilt—"

"And fear—"

"For having messed up the works—."

Both of us paused, thinking of the ramifications of what we were discussing. We could have slipped far deeper into philosophizing—it felt like every statement spawned several paths devolving into new territory.

Many times during our conversations, Dottee and I get into brain-expanding explorations, feeding thoughts off each other like balls bouncing in a handball court. I brushed that temptation aside now, as time was slipping by too fast, and I still wanted her to explain how gemstones are effective therapy.

"Moving from the esoteric to the practical, Dottee, how do gemstones work? Do they work in a similar way to color?"

We were both back to reality now. "Yes and no," she replied. "They have minerals in them, along with light. In their formation there is a mineral balance. The minerals within the gemstones have an effect on body chemistry. If you need calcium, you should wear organic gems. (By the way, radiation therapy reduces calcium in the body.) So you wear organic gemstones: shells and pearls and coral. They are calcium carbonates. Amber is petrified sap from a pine tree, and that has a reaction with the 'sap' within you.

"During my own radiation therapy I used banded gemstones. Your energy field has order. There is order in the universe. Our planetary system revolves around the sun. That's order.

"You have the exact same order in your personal universe. But when the radiation therapy comes in it blows your field apart.

"So I took gemstones that had order, linear order. They were the banded agate and the Botswana agate. They gave me the design pattern to help my energy field. I used the mineral chemistry and the design form of the gemstones, and that's how they helped me.

"A gemstone exchanges its mineral with your blood chemistry on what is called a sub-atomic level. You can't see it, but it's doing it."

I am learning just a little about this exciting new world of quantum physics. I don't pretend to understand much, but when it is explained in simple terms, I can grasp some of the concepts.

All kinds of interactions are taking place on a sub-atomic level that challenge our ideas of what matter is and how matter behaves. It seems entirely rational to me, seen in the light of quantum physics, that gemstones could exchange minerals with elements of our bodies.

Dottee has written a number of books about gems and their healing powers. The best known is *Stone Power*, published by Warner Books. Many other books about color, nutrition, and healing have issued from her prolific pen—or computer these days. They are listed, along with other books that have been helpful to me, in the "Resources" section at the end of this book.

The tape clicked off, deciding for us that we were through for now. We will never be through, really, because we continue to evolve and learn—so Dottee and I still come together from time to time to touch bases and share new awarenesses. We are living in a pretty exciting epoch, so there is a lot to share.

How did Dottee Mella help me heal? She did just what she said she would do. She helped me peel back the banana, and I was left looking at the soft inside. It has always amused me that if you stick your tongue in the middle of a round slice of banana it divides into three parts. (Try it sometime.) So it is with her therapy. The first part is seeing clearly, the second is stimulating creativity to help understand the forces that have shaped the problem and the third part is doing something about it.

You don't swallow the banana until you have chewed it.

In my case, she helped me see the major causes of disharmony between my external and internal lives. The main issues were powerlessness and lack of self love.

I had put myself in a position of servitude, she told me, when inside I was not happy to be a slave. A controlling father, a passive mother, and a society which encouraged women to be dependent were the main formative influences allowing me to be taken advantage of by men—honored to be whistled at, flattered to be a sex object, even raped; always powerless to prevent or confront.

Then I had married an angry, controlling man and was a housewife for twenty years. I raised four wonderful, vigorous children, but never worked outside the home. Not content with that level of servitude, I took in three more children. (Now that my children are grown, they all are a major source of love and support for me and they have become wonderful, contributing citizens of the world. But oh, those teen years.)

When I finally divorced, I was a "displaced homemaker"—educated, but having no work skills, no job record. How's that for powerlessness? Following my programming, I had done a good job of keeping myself that way. When I announced my intention to divorce, my mother anxiously said to me, in perfect concordance with her Victorian upbringing, "But who is going to take care of you?" That's a pretty good illustration of what the culture of my generation expected of me.

After the divorce, however, I started to take my power. I took a class in Transactional Analysis and I found a job through a government program for displaced homemakers.

Then I fell in love and found myself in a new male-female relationship. This time I married a kind man, a nurturing man. For the first time in my life I was being "cared for," and it felt wonderful. What I did not realize was the pendulum had swung the other way but the issues were the same.

I was happy, but the old problems of powerlessness, now underground, didn't go away. There are many ways to allow yourself to be controlled. Anger and fear are obvious ones, but nurturing concern, even in love, can be controlling too. Fortunately, as I walked the path of understanding, my dear husband walked the path too, beside me. We both had lessons to learn.

We had been married six years when we moved my elderly mother from her home near New York City to an apartment close to us in New Mexico. This move brought me face to face with a lot of old mother/child issues. Even if the mother is in her nineties and the daughter in her fifties, the old relationship problems are the same—but skewed, because the mother now becomes the child, while still remaining the mother. Pretty confusing.

So, because the old, belabored issues were never resolved, they came and shook me by the shoulder.

I got breast cancer.

Now I *really* had to do something about them.

Dottee helped me expose and understand the issues, then gave me tools to work on them with visualization, colors and affirmations, plus the reinforcement of her positive personal energy. I know now that it was a doorway I had to walk through, and the path to changing the old programming is a long one.

A back-to-life journey is like peeling an onion—a metaphor I was to hear often. Take a layer off and another is waiting underneath.

It's hard work. There are tears. Help is welcome. Help is necessary. Forget trying to do it all yourself. Even the Lone Ranger had Tonto.

I don't know if Dottee's prediction that I will become a healer will come true. But if anyone reading this book finds something helpful, encouraging or enlightening, then perhaps I am already performing that function.

I hope so.

Returning now to the point along the road when I had first seen Dottee, I still had to continue my own physical healing—and the next, very consuming and very physical procedure, was hiking through that "Grand Canyon" of chemotherapy.

Entering the Grand Canyon of Chemotherapy

J O H N   H .   S A I K I

The Medical Oncologist

Chugging along on this hypothetical journey, you can imagine I had left L.A. and was negotiating the coastal mountains. Some of the valleys had serious sinkholes; occasionally hillcrests allowed breathtaking views beyond. Time had warped into a puzzling blend of here, now, and eternity.

Barely more than a week had gone by since the mastectomy, yet already Ted and I were standing in the parking lot of the University of New Mexico Cancer Center, about to see my medical oncologist, Dr. Saiki, for the first time. Strange how time can be distorted. Those eight days after surgery were a blur of activity, yet every individual moment stretched into forever.

During that week I had gone home, received my pathology report, and returned to Dr. McIver to get my drains removed. We had taken my sister-in-law to the airport (my first driving trip), called the cancer hot line (1-800-4CANCER) for information, and put our personal support troops on full alert. I walked every day, visited my mother, and took care of all the little things that make up ordinary life, filling the moments until the big treatment was to begin.

Before Toni went back to Chicago she put a note on my refrigerator door, a quote from the Bible: "My grace shall be sufficient unto thee, for My strength is made perfect in weakness." Those inspiring words sustained me through many valleys and also illuminated hillcrest vistas.

Now, as we began the long walk from parking lot to Cancer Center, Ted and I held hands in mutual support, and I silently prayed those words. Going into that building felt like entering a tornado that would suck us in like Dorothy and Toto. My future, our future, seemed entirely in somebody else's hands, and that was scary.

A word about my husband. Ted tends to feel faint anywhere near hospitals. To him, ignorance is bliss when it comes to how the human body works. He doesn't want to know—-quickly turns off medical news on the television; becomes suddenly deaf, abandoning ship when conversations slip into medical waters. Being aware of this, I appreciated even more the devotion that guided him to be with me, physically and emotionally, as we approached the Cancer Center's automatic doors. A hug, a couple of deep breaths, and we passed through that gateway into the vortex.

Surprise! This was not a dark, scary place, but a bustling, efficient clinic staffed with cheerful people, much like any other doctor's offices. The patients in the waiting rooms looked like any other patients, too. What had I expected? Dull gray walls and dull gray people getting ready to die. There were plenty of patients there, all ages and all walks of life, and every one had cancer—but it didn't look like they were getting ready to die. They looked amazingly well!

After being guided through inevitable paperwork we found ourselves in Dr. Saiki's examining room. Hollow moments, each seeming an hour, passed by.

"You OK?" Ted touched my hand.

"Yeah. You?" He nodded. I knew his stomach hurt. Mine wasn't so great either. My mouth was dry and my heart pumping like an athlete running the hundred-yard dash.

Silence.

"Want to look at a magazine?" He picked up an old issue of *People* and handed it to me.

"Sure." I lied. Images of smiling movie stars and sports figures flashed into my eyes but made no connection with my brain.

More silence.

Finally Dr. Saiki entered the room and shook our hands. He was younger than I had imagined, but any other impressions were trapped in my enveloping cloud of anxiety as we watched him sift through pages of reports attached to the mysterious Ploski patient chart. What was in those pages? At last he looked up with sympathetic eyes.

"In your case I believe we should pursue an aggressive course of chemotherapy for six months, followed by five weeks of radiation therapy, followed by tamoxifen for the rest of your life. It will be hard, and there are no guarantees. If it works, great! If it doesn't, then care becomes simply palliative."

The words hit hard. I stammered. "N-no guarantees?"

"No guarantees," he repeated quietly and firmly. My heart sank. In heavy silence his words hung, echoing. I almost asked, "No hope?" but just couldn't get it out of my mouth.

Dr. Saiki went on to describe how he would treat me. I was to have a catheter implanted in a large vein near my heart, through which the chemotherapy was to be delivered. I was to have eight sessions of chemotherapy, each three weeks apart, and each lasting about three hours. The main chemical, adriamycin, was to be infused at home for two days after each chemo session, by means of a small pump attached to the catheter. My hair would fall out. My immune system would be taken to an all-time low, so I would be on high-powered antibiotics for ten days each three weeks. There was danger of irreversible heart damage, so before each session I was to have what is called a "Muga" scan to monitor heart function. Each week I would have a blood test to check on the effects of the drugs. It sounded like total commitment to the Cancer Center for half a year, and it sounded awful. I asked if everyone was treated this aggressively. Dr. Saiki told me no, but an aggressive approach was necessary in my case because so many lymph nodes were involved.

His voice became kind. "Don't hold your emotions in," he counseled. "Gather your family around you. Hold each other. Cry together." By then I had decided he is a very nice person, but he sure did lay it on the line. Niceness didn't make the fears about my prognosis or the treatment go away. I had to trust his skills and the latest in medical technology and also—I was later to find—his incredible intuition.

After making an appointment for surgery to install the catheter we left the Cancer Center. Both of us were pretty depressed. There wasn't much to say, so the forty-minute ride back home was a quiet one. Just some hand holding and hugs at traffic stops, my head on Ted's shoulder, silent tears prickling behind closed eyes.

I reluctantly telephoned the results to mother, friends and children, who were concerned and supportive. But we were never able to take Dr. Saiki's advice and sit down together and cry. We felt awful, but strong programming kicked in. We tried not to let each other and the rest of the world see our internal anguish. "Don't feel sorry for yourself," the programming repeated endlessly. "Be strong. Don't make others feel bad." What garbage!

Fortunately, it was that very afternoon Dottee Mella came over and my spirits got a much-needed boost. Listening to Dottee restored my balance. By the time I went to bed, sleep, my precious escape from reality, came as a welcome friend. Oddly, I never had any nightmares. Reality was nightmare enough!

Two days later we went to the University of New Mexico Hospital, physically connected to the Cancer Center, for a Muga scan. Ted led me through a maze of unfamiliar corridors.

"Should we leave a trail of bread crumbs?" Gallows humor. He laughed a gallows laugh. Finally the waiting room came into view, and we both sat down by a large tank full of busy fish to await the technician's call.

This test, like the bone scan, uses nuclear medicine. First they inject you with a nuclear substance that has a half-life of a day or so. They assure you that you are not radioactive (but warn you not to go near pregnant women. Huh?) Then back to the seat by the fish tank for about twenty minutes, while the nuclear material goes through your circulatory system. At that point another injection of a substance teams up with the nuclear stuff to make your pumping heart visible. Immediately, they put you up on a gurney, paste on electrodes and ask you to lie still while they position this monster camera right up against your chest wall.

"Breathe normally," says the technician, and you breathe as normally as you can while the camera takes pictures of your heart in action. On the room's far wall, another technician manipulates a bank of computers and video screens that show your heart doing its thing. It's weird and a little scary to see that going on inside you, so I close my eyes. They freeze-frame specific shots and call out numbers and it's all very mysterious, but it doesn't hurt. Throughout the chemotherapy this process was repeated every three weeks, just before chemo was administered, to make sure adriamycin was not damaging my heart. After a while, the receptionist, technicians and fish got to know Ted and me pretty well. I even relaxed to the point of being able to breathe normally, or almost normally.

As I came out of the Muga scan treatment room that first day, Ted's eyes asked the question.

"It wasn't so bad," I reassured him. "Piece of cherry pie!" I really was relieved, even to the point of joking about how I could light up a flashlight with residual nuclear radiation. Or worse, light him up. I growled and approached him menacingly, arms extended.

"Oh no!" he faked terror, running away from me down our imaginary trail of bread crumbs back to the Cancer Center.

There, Catherine the surgical nurse showed us a video about the Groshong catheter. We saw happy, healthy looking people going about their daily tasks with no indication that under their blouses tubes protruded from their chests and snaked under the skin into their veins. It all looked so easy. Even Ted watched the surgical procedure without blanching. It's extraordinary how the media can sugar-coat something when there is a product to hype!

There were six days to wait until the "minor" operation to install that catheter. I did a lot of thinking and lifestyle changing. Of course, true to my nature, I went full steam ahead; soaking grains and eating them raw, taking herbs and supplements, reading about alternative therapies. I told Ted to get ready for anything weird I was about to undertake, because I was going to do everything possible to help myself. My husband isn't too fond of things he can't see or hear, feel, taste or smell; and he was suspicious of non-traditional healing therapies—but I think he was so scared for me, and so supportive, that he agreed to anything I proposed to do, as long as I kept walking the allopathic path at the Cancer Center. As time went on, he learned a lot from all my healers too.

The day after the Muga scan my doorbell rang. Betty, a "Reach to Recovery" woman from the American Cancer Society, sailed in like the figurehead on an old clipper ship. She was stunning! White hair, beautifully coifed, Black Watch tartan skirt and white blouse covering what seemed to be two generously sized normal breasts. A youthful face and vigorous body belied her sixty-five years. This was a cancer survivor!

"Cynthia," as she checked me off her list of people to see that day, "I am here to show you how to regain full use of your arm and give you a soft breastform to wear until you get your permanent prosthesis. You can't use a silicone one yet—it's too soon after surgery. Silicone breastforms are heavy, made that way so that they can hang down at the same latitude as your real breast. I got a new one recently and I'm really happy with it."

I looked at the two matching breasts under her blouse. I couldn't see any difference between them. "Which one is it?"

She told me.

"Would you mind if I touch it?"

"Not at all. You'll see it feels very natural."

So I gingerly pressed her fake breast and found it felt pretty normal. That was encouraging, because although I had consulted a plastic surgeon about reconstructive surgery, I was loathe to put my body through any more than it was already enduring. Later, the silicone breast implant controversy erupted, confirming my decision.

We sat down to a cup of herb tea, while she filled out some forms for the American Cancer Society. Then she began to teach me.

"Cynthia, you have to exercise your arm every day to keep it from tightening up, by holding on to the top of a door, reaching into kitchen cabinets, anything that will extend the arm. Gradually reach higher and higher."

"How long will I have to do this?"

She smiled, ruefully. "Always. Forever." She brought out a gadget that hooks on top of a door, with two strings hanging down from it. We put it on top of a bedroom door and she demonstrated how to hold the strings with both hands and pull them, one at a time, to stretch the hand up the door. I could only get within a foot of the top.

"A gift from the American Cancer Society," she told me as she placed the gadget on the table. The other gift was a nylon tricot breast shaped pocket which she stuffed with absorbent cotton.

"Here's your new breast for a while." I thanked her, grateful for at least a bulge to offset my newly boyish, but very lopsided, figure.

"Would you mind telling me about your breast cancer?" I asked. She seemed so open, and I was interested to hear her story. Why had she done so well?

"Well," Betty began, "Eight years ago they gave me up as impossible to cure. It was very serious. But they put me through chemotherapy, radiation, and I am still on tamoxifen, and that was eight years ago! I went through it all."

"How did you feel? Were you scared?"

"Sure, I was scared, but I'm a golfer, and I was determined not to let it get me down. So I was playing golf two weeks after surgery, and have stayed busy and active ever since."

"Did your hair fall out?"

"Oh yes, my hair fell out, and it made me mad because it was summertime, and I still wanted to play golf. It was really hot, so I put ice cubes under my wig and teed off. That worked pretty well, but then the ice cubes melted and I had water running down my face!" She laughed at the memory.

I enjoyed our conversation. It was full of little tips, woman to woman. She showed me a mastectomy bra and told me of the American Cancer Society services. Her vigor, humor and warmth—and obvious good health—were so encouraging! Just the right person to motivate the newly vulnerable! I basked in borrowed energy long after her departure. Her prognosis had been as bad as mine but she had beat it! What a role model! That very afternoon I took mother downtown shopping, and I bought a mastectomy bra. A step forward. Words cannot express the lift that vibrant cancer survivor gave me. I'll always be grateful.

I was beginning to understand how deeply other people affected me, and how much courage I could gain from them. They helped me get up enough nerve to start sailing my own ship. There was something I wanted, so I told Dr. Saiki about it. I wanted to go to New York City before I started chemotherapy, to do something very special. I wanted to attend a Broadway opening.

My children all live in different states, so we don't have many opportunities to get together. Melanie, the oldest, who is a nurse, was living in California at that time. She and her husband, John, had a little girl, Emilie. Since then, baby Douglas has joined the family.

Jim was an airline executive. He and his wife Ellen, and their daughters Cassie and Jessica, reside in the Phoenix area.

Alissa, a talented dressmaker, was living in Houston with husband Phil and daughters Karinne and Noelle.

Michael, the youngest, a dancer/singer/actor, parked his body anywhere his job took him. Right then, it took him to New York City, where he was about to make his Broadway debut as a featured dancer in "Fiddler on the Roof," starring the legendary Topol.

Michael's debut felt like a pretty big family deal, so all my children were going to get together to attend the opening. I was determined to be there too. Dr. Saiki said, "Great! We encourage people to keep excitement in their lives. We'll delay starting the chemotherapy until the day after you get back."

It seemed like a good way to put chemotherapy out of my mind for a while; but before leaving, I still had to get that catheter implanted in my chest.

So once again I got ready for surgery. They call it minor surgery, but to my way of thinking any time they cut into you and poke around, it is major. Especially if they are fooling around with the vein that leads directly into your heart.

Breakfastless again, I presented myself at the UNM hospital. This time the surgeon was a trauma surgeon. He is very good at what he does. This is what Catherine tells me as we wait for him to enter the little operating room. She also tells me why I cannot be sedated. I need to be able to tell them if anything feels wrong, or peculiar. I am not reassured. Nervously, I start counting ceiling tiles from my position on an operating table.

"Don't worry, he's really very good. He's the only one that inserts the Groshong catheter. He does a lot of them."

This also does not reassure me. We wait some more. Nervousness is not diminishing. Catherine has scrubbed and sterilized my chest and covered it up. Thin cotton drapes may keep out germs, but they are not much of a buffer against the coolness of the room. I shiver, and resume counting ceiling tiles.

She brings a blanket to cover my lower half, and then goes to see what is keeping him. He is held up by a complication from some other surgery. That's not exactly comforting news, but I try to develop a positive attitude. I start all over on the disrupted tile count.

Finally the surgeon comes in, all business. Definitely not Mr. Personality. He gives me an injection to deaden the insertion site, then cuts me there on the remaining breast a couple inches below the heart and runs a wire under the skin up to my collar bone. He is fast and he is rough. It hurts. The wire makes a funny crunching sound as it moves through the flesh. I feel like a small child, helpless and abused. Catherine reaches under the sheet and grabs my hand, holding tight. Gratitude floods me at this simple gesture of support. I will never cease to appreciate her compassion.

He makes another incision just above the collar bone and runs the catheter down the tunnel to my breast again, and sticks the other end in the vena cava, that big vein feeding the heart. A couple of stitches to close the sites and he leaves the room. I am lying there with a tube hanging from my breast, a sutured vampire bite on the neck; trembling, feeling like a wounded bird, wings broken, unable to fly.

"You did just fine." Catherine pats me on the shoulder and wheels me out to where Ted is waiting. The two of them roll me down to X-ray, where they take pictures to be sure the catheter is in the right place. I am weeping quietly. Dr. Saiki confirms it was done correctly. Catherine gives me supplies and instructions for care of the catheter, and helps me into the car Ted has brought up from the parking lot. As bad as I feel at that moment, I still know wild buffalo wouldn't stop me from getting on that plane to New York City, three days later.

There weren't any wild buffalo; it was bladder spasms the next day that almost did me in. Another quick trip to the Cancer Center, an antibiotic prescription from Dr. Saiki, and I was ready to go again. Who can doubt the effect of stress on the bladder?

The next anxiety was airport security. What would they think of all my equipment? The hypodermic needles and vials of saline solution needed for daily catheter flushing were in my suitcase, which also contained bags of vitamins, enzymes and herbs. I must not fit the profile of a drug courier, however, for they didn't ask any questions, just passed me through.

On the airplane at last, my children around me, I began to relax. I still felt pretty fragile. What a comfort to have my daughter/nurse along!

Somewhere over the prairie I pulled out a tape Mary Carroll Nelson had given me. It was Deepak Chopra, M.D., addressing a meeting of holistic physicians. As I listened to that tape, a whole new picture of the nature of disease and healing emerged. Chopra, a renowned Boston endocrinologist, gave up the practice of western medicine to embrace his Ayurvedic medical heritage. He began treating people according to thousands of years old Ayurvedic practices, and he found they were getting well.

This is an exciting time to be alive, as quantum physics is giving us a whole new understanding of the mechanics of matter and life. Traditionally disparate views of science and religion are beginning to weave together. At long last, knowledge that has been held by mystics for eons is being supported by science. What clearly emerges is that our

perceptions of everything are formed by the early patterning of our surroundings. Our belief systems create what is real to us. Conversely, by
changing our belief systems, we can influence our reality to change.
Chopra supports the interrelationship of all aspects of our selves—
mind, emotions, body, soul—believing that wellness depends on balance and harmony among them all.

Chopra's tape gave me a sense of power, of control over my own
destiny, based on awareness and choice. I would never feel so helpless
again! I see that tape as a hilltop vista in my learning journey, a gateway
to new ways of understanding myself and the universe. By the time the
plane landed in Newark, I had moved up intellectually to a new plateau.

The whole bunch of us were welcomed warmly by my dear friend-
for-life Karol Teiko, who opened her home and heart to us. Karol had
been my roommate for two years at Middlebury College in Vermont,
back in the early 1950s. We had lost track of each other for more than
thirty years, until one day my phone rang and there was Karol. What joy
to recover that lost friendship! Now she and her husband Jesse were
sharing this special occasion with all of us.

The memory of that weekend will always stand out in Technicolor.
Golden days, love of family and friends, feasting in Karol and Jesse's
cozy kitchen, picture taking in the warm autumn sunshine, walking in
the red, yellow and russet leaves.

And then there was the excitement of the Broadway opening; the
thrill of seeing Michael as a Russian dancing with Topol, and Michael
as a Jew playing the cymbals and singing that heart-catching music. A
fantastic cast flawlessly performed the funny/sad story that has moved
two generations to laughter and to tears. It was fun attending the cast
party afterwards, and meeting members of the cast and Broadway
celebrities. By the time we all stumbled onto the plane Sunday morning
I was too tired to even think of the first chemotherapy session coming
up Tuesday morning.

But Tuesday morning did arrive, and I did enter the Grand Canyon
of chemotherapy. Stepped off the rim and began walking the difficult
Kaibab trail to the bottom. Six months later I began the climb back up
and resumed my journey towards the light.

Dr. Saiki had armed me with a bunch of prescriptions. There was
medicine to help me sleep, medicine to take away nausea, medicine to
keep my blood from clotting too much, medicine to avoid infections.

There is no doubt he made every effort to ease me through the process, to give me as much comfort as possible.

I want to make it clear that not all chemotherapy is as difficult as mine was. There are other, milder forms of cancer-killing drugs, and on the other hand there is something known as "high dose" chemotherapy that is even tougher. People on that program must be hospitalized for treatment, scrupulous care taken to avoid infection— even to the point of a prohibition against eating raw food. Dr. Saiki was giving me what he called an "aggressive" course of therapy. What that means is the next step down from an atomic bomb. I received a computer printout of what he considers to be "aggressive" therapy. When the bills started coming in, I found that he had far exceeded the doses on that printout. The theory is, in a serious case like mine, "Give her all she can take." They judge how much you can handle by keeping track of your white blood cell count—a measure of immune system function. They administer enough to bring the white count down from an average of 5,000-7,000 to under 1,000. Then they wait three weeks for you to make enough new white blood cells to do it all over again. Nobody knows how a patient will tolerate chemotherapy the first time it is given, so new patients are watched especially carefully.

I must also make it very clear here that every patient is different. There are many specialized kinds of chemotherapy. But even when the same protocol is administered, individual patients will react different- ly. What follows here is simply my own story—the truth of what hap- pened to me. I hope it contains information that will be helpful to other people, but the purpose is not to give medical advice. The read- er should not assume it is exactly the same for everybody, and should always rely on the advice of his or her physician.

Anyway, that first day I ate breakfast before going to the Cancer Center. Not a good idea to do this on an empty stomach, I was told. On the way there I plugged into my Walkman and listened to Bernie Siegel's tape "Preparing for Chemotherapy." He said things like "See the medicine as helping you. ...Don't see it as harming you. ...Know that it is indeed effective. ...Make it your friend. ...Visualize it killing cancer cells." Psyching me up. *Ready or not, here I come! All-y All- y In-free!*

By this time the path from the parking lot to the Cancer Center was very familiar. Plum trees lining the walk were losing their autumn leaves that day. Before the full course of treatment was over, I saw bare branches in winter, beautiful pink blossoms in spring, and glossy mahogany leaves in summer. They counted time passing towards my release.

Inside the Center, Bev, a chemo nurse, came to attend me. I was expecting a gentle, soft-spoken person who would allay my fears. Instead, this bustling, compact mover and shaker grabbed my arm propelling me down the hall, amusing people in the waiting rooms by exclaiming in an embarrassingly loud voice, "First time? A-ha! *A virgin!*"— Evil laugh— "Come with me, my pretty. Ha, ha, ha..."

Over her shoulder, "You can come back for her in about three hours." Ted stood there looking uncertain. "Don't worry, we won't lose her!" With Bev, there was no turning back. We were already far down the hall.

She steered me into a small room that looked sort of like a dentist's office. Two high form-fitting chairs, each one attended by an intravenous hookup pole, dominated the space. Little handmade crafty stuff decorated mirrors and walls.

"Hang your jacket over there and climb on up. Get comfortable. I see you brought a Walkman. What are you listening to? Rock? Rap? Grateful Dead?"

"Golden Voyages. It's real soothing."

"I don't know that one. We have some other tapes here for people who want to listen to them instead of my golden voice."

What could I say? Bev was totally in charge. She bustled around, arranging a tray of paraphernalia, joshing and nattering. It's not my style, but I couldn't help liking her, and soon she had me nattering back. She hung a bag of red liquid on the pole, arranged the I-V lines and stuck the needle into the rubber cap on the end of my catheter. As liquid started dripping through the catheter, I felt coolness entering my chest.

"That's just saline solution, to be sure the catheter isn't clogged," she explained. "Then we put in some joy juice—otherwise known as ativan—to make you happy, and when you wake up it's all over. Do you want a blanket?"

She brought a hand-knit afghan about the size of a crib blanket. I adjusted the Walkman and began listening to soft melodies rising over a babbling brook. My hands and feet started feeling antsy, so I kicked off my shoes and shook out my hands. Eyes drooped closed, ears slow-ly melted into that Golden Voyage…and I woke up to see Bev hooking up a pump the size and shape of a basting syringe to the catheter.

"You're all done. Just wear this inside your shirt for twenty-four hours, and then when it's empty replace it with this other one. The pump works by your body heat to deliver the adriamycin over forty-eight hours. It's safer that way. Call us if you have any problems, and we'll see you in a week for a blood test."

That wasn't so bad, I thought. And then I tried to stand up. Bev caught me as I slid down from the chair. She supported me while I staggered out into the hall, giddy and feeling slightly drunk, plopped me in a wheel chair, pushed me out the automatic doors and bundled me into the car Ted had brought up.

"I feel fine. I feel like eating a hamburger."

"Sure, honey."

Not much of the trip home comes back to mind, or any of the other subsequent trips home after chemotherapy. Each time, when we got home, Ted would undress me and pour me into bed, where I sank back into oblivion for a number of hours.

Dr. Saiki is merciful. In addition to the chemotherapeutic agents, he directs that analgesics, anti-nausea drugs and anti-inflammatory drugs be administered with the chemo. I really did feel good, if physically sloppy, after the chemo session; and the lack of nausea surprised me. Until midnight, when I threw up—just once—so that wasn't too bad.

Next day the body felt pretty good, but the mind kept forgetting things. "That's the ativan," Melanie told me on the phone. I did some laundry, wrote letters and futzed around the house, noting all the while little side effects like tingling scalp and minor diarrhea.

For a few days I felt kind of nauseated, like being newly pregnant, but compasine took care of it. I was not incapacitated. During the next couple of weeks, Ted and I were able to get out and walk on the mesa. I took little walks by myself. I had to rest a lot, but managed to keep moving pretty well. One treatment down, seven more to go! I was to find they became harder as time went on.

Over the next few months I got weaker, but never to the point where I had to stay in bed. Our walks became shorter, our outings fewer as winter closed in and I sank into the structure of this protocol. Every evening around five o'clock the big brown recliner welcomed my body.

I would pull up a blanket and Ted and I would watch TV with dogs and cats on our laps, comforting us with their love.

At the worst point, near the end of chemotherapy, I could only walk about two hundred yards. My hands were so weak I couldn't grip a nail clipper to cut my nails, and the muscles in my legs were so stiff that I couldn't sit on the floor. Had it not been for acupuncture, I think I would have been in bed. By then, I had begun my "other" healing therapies, and I am convinced they helped see me through. More on them later.

Over time, I became aware of a pattern in the effects of each course of chemo. Notes from my journal:

Day 1 — Chemotherapy. Groggy.

Day 2 — Still feel groggy, but OK.

Day 3 — Feel nauseated. Need composine several times. Finish adriamycin pump.

Day 4 — Feel better. Appetite returns. Want saltines, popcorn, Ted's famous mashed potatoes.

Day 5 — Feel pretty good.

Day 6 — Feel pretty good.

Day 7 — Start to feel woozy, dizzy when moving too fast. Blood pressure falls.

Day 8 — Esophagus starts to burn. Mouth sores. Diarrhea. Sore rectum.

Days 9 20   General malaise, but gradual recovery. Third week, feel pretty good.

Day 21 - Start all over again.

Chemotherapy was the structure of my life for six long months. Halfway through, Melanie sent me a half dozen white roses. At the end, she sent a dozen. I still have them. Their dried petals are affixed one by one to my art, incorporating that healing energy into the work.

Several incidents stand out in that blur of time. Losing my hair was one of them. Two weeks after the first chemo I was drying off in the shower when I noticed one very long pubic hair hanging down. I pulled on it, and it came out easily, along with a bunch of others! Then as I dried my hair, a nest of gray and brown/blond decorated the towel. I took to wearing a turban to bed, because every morning there would be globs of hair on the pillow. One day, walking on the mesa with Ted, I pulled out a hank of it and hung it on a juniper tree for the birds to use. From then on I saved it in a pink plastic bag every day and when the bag was full I went back on the mesa and ceremonially decorated the tree. It was getting close to Christmas. Merry Christmas, birds!

HAIR! What an important part of our self image! We have fussed with it, crimped, curled, frizzed and straightened it, dyed it, cut it, grown it, agonized over it. Plays have been written about it, lockets filled with it. In humiliation and mourning hair is shorn. Ancient Indians used women's hair for ropes—the men grew hair long. Delilah sapped Sampson's strength by cutting it. Many things can be done to it—but not when you don't have any.

Bald is not beautiful. Looking in the mirror, an unfamiliar image peered back. Ugly. Ugh-lee! Shiny, soft scalp, aging face, unembellished. Losing hair is a real challenge to your sense of self. It's hard to see yourself as beautiful, even inside your heart, when the glare of a bald head blinds your eyes. How silly it seems for people to get distressed that their hair doesn't look just right—they are lucky to even have any! And what a miracle that it just *grows,* unseeded, unwatered, on top of heads!

Hair may be considered beautiful or ugly, but in the most practical sense, it's there to protect your head from cold, heat and sunburn. It was winter, and my head was cold. Our neighbor Grace crocheted me a turquoise green cap, and I had a pink turban. They covered my baldness day and night. The wig was scratchy and uncomfortable, so it was worn only outside the house.

Another special event I remember was the day I was working at my drawing board and a show featuring John Bradshaw came on the TV. It caught my interest. He was talking about the hurts we all endured as children, and how they affect our life as adults. He was telling people to nurture the child within themselves, give it love, discover the hurts, get them out and let them go. People were crying and hitting pillows—it got pretty intense, but something in me was hooked.

So I decided to use art to heal the child in my heart. I started a series of left-hand drawings about my childhood. Wow! They were not pretty! There was big father (I scribbled red all over him), mother, sister and me, all little. There was the dirty old sea captain who molested me. I colored him black and gave him dripping fangs! I poured all my emotions into the pictures, in words and colors. They were far from pretty pictures, they were horror stories! Ted looked at them, scattered over the studio floor.

"You going to burn these? I don't like them." Ted the peacemaker, fugitive from anger, was disturbed that such ugliness was in me and could be expressed. I was kind of surprised at the ugliness too, since I prefer to think of myself as a nice person, but letting all that out was a catharsis. Little Cynthia within had screamed out those bad feelings and now I could hold her close to my heart and soothe her.

"Yeah, but I want to take slides of them first, in case someone else can use them." But before doing so, I drew another, of me holding my inner child. This one was peaceful. I felt lighter.

Still, as if some evil thing lurked behind me, ready to pounce, every night I resumed a battle with fear and depression. Every ache was a possible metastasis. Every time I dried off from the shower my body got a paranoid once-over to check for lumps or bumps. And the weekly trips to get blood drawn, plus the chemo sessions, reinforced that insecurity. After all, cancer clinics are not wellness centers! They are treatment centers for sick people. Going there reminds you of your illness, not your health.

Another event was that sometime early in the course of treatment, before the second chemo, the catheter refused to donate blood for a weekly blood test.

"Don't worry" said Joe, the friendly, cheerful laboratory boss, "It's probably positional. Raise your arms." Still no blood.

"Lean forward" No dice. It just won't issue forth.

"Let's try you lying on your side." He called to his pretty assistant, "Vicky, help Cynthia over to the table, please."

Vicky took my arm and eased me up on a table, giving me a little pat on the shoulder and an encouraging smile. Eventually a little blood trickled into the syringe and we cheered.

That was only the beginning of my catheter troubles, however. Each week it became harder to get blood. We tried every position I was capable of. As a last resort, still hoping it was positional—lodged against the vein wall—Bev the expert was called in to turn me upside down, slap my back, and engineer every peculiar inverted position I could manage. When that didn't work, it became apparent that the problem was not positional; I was clotting up the tube. We tried heparin, then streptokinase. Week after week it became more of a struggle to produce blood for testing.

There were times I was glad for that catheter, though. For instance, one morning I woke up feeling rotten. Cold and flu rotten, not chemo rotten. By the time I saw Dr. Saiki for an emergency appointment in the afternoon I was running a temperature of 103°. This is a definite no-no when you are on chemo, as the immune system, your defense against infection, is crippled. Saiki ordered liquid penicillin immediately, intravenously through the catheter; then afterwards he stood looking at me and Ted, his mind busy with possible courses of action.

"I ordinarily would hospitalize you immediately," he mused, (sinking sensation in my stomach) "but somehow I have a feeling you will do OK at home. Bev can show you how to administer the bags of liquid penicillin, and you can call me immediately if you feel worse." (Joy! I dreaded being hospitalized.)

Dr. Saiki's intuition was right on target. Once a day for three days I hung the bag of penicillin from the bedroom door and hooked it up to my catheter—and I got better real fast. The catheter was my life line that time.

Weeks crawled by. After the third chemo I started getting quite a lot weaker. Spent a lot of time in meditation, made good friends with my Angel, talked a lot to God and Divine Mother. Moved into the spare bedroom, comforting my aching muscles on the warm water bed, napped daily, listened to music, turned inward.

As always, a move inward was balanced with a move outward. I wrote up a list of techniques that were helping me deal with the side effects of chemotherapy and gave them to my oncologist to offer new patients.

And yet I was slipping, physically and emotionally, into a sort of resignation that was dangerous.

One morning I got a call from my psychic friend and healer Celesta Meola, who lives in Yardley, Pennsylvania.

"Cynthia," she announced in imperative tones, "You and I met on the Astral Plane last night and I read you the riot act!"

"What? Come on."

"We met on the Astral Plane," she reaffirmed, "and I told you that you had better get your energy flowing in a positive direction. You are slipping, and you need to rev up."

"Celesta, I feel so tired and lousy. And I just got over a cold."

"That explains it! You were cold when I met you last night, and I told you never to come up there again without a coat!" We laughed at the pun, knowing that's sometimes the way information is transferred.

"I know you feel lousy," she continued, "but you can move forward. You have to move forward. Make yourself a five-year plan and know that you are going to be here to accomplish it."

A five year plan? What a thought! Here I was wondering if I was going to be alive in a few months. But I knew Celesta well, and trusted her. She had always felt that I would be OK. Anyway, it made sense to think positively. So I did make a five-year plan. I planned to buy a computer, take a correspondence course in writing children's literature and build our dream house in Colorado. That was five years ago. I didn't finish the correspondence course, but instead this book is being written on my new computer and we have finalized house plans, brought in electricity and water, and are in the process of building. It sure feels good.

That five year-plan was a landmark in my recovery. There were still a lot of obstacles, however—like that catheter. After the fourth chemotherapy session I went home as usual, adriamycin pump attached. The next day, after changing the pump to the second dose I had a terrible coughing fit, followed by a bad ache in the neck and chest area. Soon, redness and burning appeared under the skin along the track of the catheter. The adriamycin was backing up along the track! The next day it got worse and I started to run a low-grade fever, so I went back to the Cancer Center. Dr. Saiki was very upset. He said it had never happened to any of his patients before. He and Catherine sat with me in his office and discussed various options. They decided to send me down to X-ray for a flow study to see what was blocking the adriamycin from entering my vein. What they found was that a blood clot had formed around the end of the catheter just inches from my heart. That sounded scary. What if it broke off and went into my heart?

Then they decided to put me on a heparin pump and send me home for a week, to see if the clot would dissolve. A visiting nurse came to my house that night and hooked me up to a pump in a fanny pack. It startled me with a funny sound every once in a while, like a crow calling far away. It slept on the pillow next to my head and got wrapped up in plastic when I bathed, but we never became good friends. I didn't like being attached to it.

A week later, another flow study showed the clot still there, so Dr. Saiki told me I would either have to stay on the pump for three more months, or else pull out the catheter. I voted to pull the catheter and suggested coming to the Cancer Center for three days in a row during each course of chemo, so that the dose of adriamycin would be administered in smaller increments over a longer period of time. That very afternoon, when I left the Cancer Center, I no longer had a catheter hanging out of my chest, and I was really glad. No more daily cleansing routine, no more sleeping in a shirt to keep from pulling on it, no more taping it to my breast! From then on the chemo would be injected into the veins in my hands.

By now I was halfway through chemotherapy. Each course left me weaker. My muscles were stiff and sore, my joints ached, I had trouble using my right thumb and my arms and legs were weak and wobbly. I had to nap every day. Nevertheless, I was able to keep up with the essentials of living: cooking, bathing, washing clothes, paying bills, and struggling with the complexities of medical insurance (which I was very grateful I had). This whole procedure is horribly expensive.

Along the way, I was finding other therapies that helped bolster my energy to keep me from being wiped out. I was fighting in every way I could, and on every level, but I had periods of depression. There were times I was not nice to my mother and long-suffering husband. I missed seeing my grandchildren, for being near them was too dangerous for my immune system. I went to the store at night, when other people were not apt to be around. I kept my distance from everyone because they might be sick. Dr. Saiki was right—it was not easy.

Boy, did I wish for a sign, a miracle.

I got one.

I no longer belong to any organized religion, but I have firm faith in the Divine, and now I felt drawn to Mary, who appeared daily for the past eleven years to a group of young people in Medjugorje, Yugoslavia. I read books about the apparitions, I prayed to her, I said the Rosary. I bought a videotape about Medjugorje and a couple of audio tapes recorded in the church there. The tapes lulled me to sleep at night, and I prayed that she would heal me. The evening before Easter Sunday I was especially down emotionally. I lay in bed listening to the music from Medjugorje and asked tearfully, "Mary, you promised you would help those who asked you. Well, I am asking!" A half-sleep came over me, and suddenly my legs from the knees down became flushed with warmth. Then a very strong, unmistakable electric current slowly tingled from my feet, up my legs, up my entire body and out my head. There was not any doubt about what was happening. In no way was it imaginary. It was vivid. It was real! I wrote in my journal:

"I feel that I have been healed, though I must go through the rest of the treatments in order to experience them and therefore be better able to serve others by sharing information. I still feel pain and the effects of chemotherapy—but that is not what the healing was for." Later I realized that my miracle occurred about the time that Easter Sunday was dawning in Medjugorje.

By the end of April I had my last chemotherapy. Betty Rice, Mary Carroll Nelson and I went out to lunch to celebrate. Bev pasted a gold star on the bandage where she pulled out the last chemo needle and declared me graduated.

"Bet you're glad to see me leave," I said.

"Yes," she acknowledged, but there's always someone new coming along." Sadly, this is true. For me, however, there was a sense of relief. I was finishing my climb back up the Kaibab Trail and heaving myself over the rim. There were to be a couple of weeks off before starting radiation therapy, and I was looking forward to the time away from the Cancer Center. "Piece of Cake," Dottee Mella had called radiation therapy. I sure hoped so.

CONVERSATION WITH DR. SAIKI

John Saiki is a small, quick, intense man with a youthful face and intelligent brown—almost black—eyes. He grew up in North Dakota, where he took the first two years of medical school at the University of North Dakota. His last two years were completed at McGill University in Montreal. He then entered the Public Health Service to fulfill his military obligation. They stationed him at Fort Defiance, Arizona. There, the visiting chairman of the University of New Mexico Department of Medicine asked him if he would like to come to Albuquerque to complete his training in internal medicine.

By that time he had decided he liked living in the southwest, so he canceled plans to complete his training at the Mayo Clinic and instead went to the University of New Mexico. While at UNM, his mentor asked him if he would be interested in setting up a leukemia/lymphoma program. He was, so he went to a famous cancer treatment center, M.D. Anderson Hospital in Houston, to learn more about chemotherapy of leukemia and lymphoma. He joined the University of New Mexico in 1970. One of his first patients was the wife of a professor of mathematics who had advanced metastatic breast cancer.

"I didn't know anything about breast cancer," he said, but he obtained outside consultation and treated her, following an unfamiliar protocol. She was very, very sick, but amazingly she started to improve—from being bedridden to using a wheelchair, to a cane and finally to walking unaided. That impressed him. As the research group associated with the University evolved, Saiki evolved with it, increasing his knowledge of treating solid tumors. Now about two-thirds of his patients are breast cancer victims. In addition to his busy clinical practice, Saiki teaches hematology and oncology at the University of New Mexico, and does clinical research as well.

Dr. Saiki's office looks like it needs to have a garage sale. There is barely room for a couple of chairs, a table and a computer amid the sheaves of papers, shelves of books and Important Clutter. The first time I ever poked my head in there I was impressed by the shelf bearing scores of rocks, fossils and interesting antiquities. Rocks, fossils and interesting antiquities are some of my favorite things, so I figured as a person he must be OK.

His office may be cluttered, but his brain is clear as crystal. He is the busiest man I know, but if someone comes in and asks him about a case, he never needs to refer to a chart. It's all there in his head.

The day I came to interview him, he was busily involved, as always. Phone to ear, he waved me to the only other chair and kept talking. I picked some papers off the seat, adding them to a pile on the table, then pulled out my notes and tape recorder. A nurse poked her head in the doorway, saw he was busy and left. I waited.

Finally he put down the phone and closed the door. He was all mine. So we got right down to it, not wanting to waste precious time.

"Dr. Saiki, this book is basically my own journey, and it's breast cancer, so although I know you deal with many other kinds, I'm only going to ask you about breast cancer. What kinds of treatments do you have available?"

He leaned forward, looking at me intently. "Whenever the disease is very localized, the treatment is basically local too. If it's extremely early, meaning there is cancer but no evidence of invasion, we just use surgery, with no radiation. If it's invasive cancer, you have to combine surgery with radiation, or more radical surgery, depending on how the woman feels about it. If there is significant risk of having recurrent tumor, meaning that there is a high likelihood of having cancer cells already spread to other parts of her body, you have to give chemotherapy in addition to surgery and radiation. And then there are hormone treatments for cancer."

"Tell me about those."

"Interestingly," he began, "when many people think about cancer they think about something like tuberculosis, something from outside that invades the body. But cancer is basically a disease of normal body cells, where the normal cells change in their behavior. Just as children can be born with abnormalities, body cells can be born with abnormalities, a multitude of them. One of these abnormalities is called cancer. But they still resemble their parent cells. If this happens to be in the breast, the breast cancer cell will resemble its normal parent breast cell. Because breast tissue will develop with the influence of female hormones, then some breast cancers can be stimulated by female hormones."

"OK, you are talking about estrogen."

"That's right. And so if you take female hormones away from a prepubertal girl, she will not develop breast tissue. We find that with roughly a third of breast cancer patients if you take away the female hormone or block it with a blocker you can cause the tumor to regress. There are other hormones that will cause it to regress, too."

I nodded my understanding. "So now what you are talking about is tamoxifen."

"Tamoxifen is a blocker," he agreed, "but progesterone, another female hormone, can cause breast cancer to regress too. There are also synthetic androgens, synthetic male hormones that have a minimal masculinizing effect, but that retain an anti-breast-cancer effect."

I had been unaware that male hormones had any effect on breast cancer, and wondered what that "minimal masculinizing effect" would be. But Dr. Saiki was on a roll.

"And then there are some other hormonal agents. Estrogen is synthesized in the ovaries, but also in the adrenal glands. So men have estrogen too ... and by the way, did you know that the biggest source for estrogen used in treating women is from the male horse, the stallion? That's because they produce so much estrogen."

"Wow!" I thought it was synthetic. But if it comes from horses, wouldn't you think it would be from the female?

"Now, what are the specific chemicals you use in chemotherapy for breast cancer?"

"The major standard adjuvant (supplemental or auxiliary) chemotherapy drugs are cytoxan, methotrexate and 5-Fluorouracil. That's standard. But if a woman has a more aggressive or more advanced tumor, then that standard adjuvant therapy is not likely to have a big enough impact. In that setting I tend to be a lot more aggressive, and I give a drug called adriamycin (that has a lot more toxicity as well), big doses of cytoxan and big doses of 5-Fluorouracil as well."

I stirred uncomfortably in my chair as I remembered my own experience with that "aggressive" program. But I felt gratitude too, because I was past it, I was here, and I was healthy.

"Exactly how do these chemicals kill cancer cells, Dr. Saiki?"

"There are different mechanisms. Probably the biggest impact is affecting the proliferation of cells. It affects the division of a malignant cell by attacking DNA. It prevents DNA from being synthesized, or binds it up somehow, or actually damages the DNA so the cell can't reproduce."

"But doesn't that do the same thing to normal cells?"

He nodded. "It does, except interestingly, normal cells have a capacity to recover and repair themselves. Cancer cells don't have that kind of ability—so they are a little more vulnerable, a little more sensitive to the chemotherapy drugs.

"Actually, cancer cells typically proliferate more slowly than normal cells. Normal cells recover very quickly, and cancer cells more slowly. When you give the next course of chemotherapy, the normal cells have recovered fully and the cancer cells have not. So the next course of chemotherapy knocks them down further."

This was news to me. I thought cancer cells reproduced wildly and out of control. I told him so.

"Yes, it sounds like wild proliferation, but it's not at all that. Although you can have an aggressive, aggressive, aggressive tumor, cancer is not likely to be a disease of rapid proliferation.

"It's more a disease where the tumor cells have forgotten how to mature. Normal cells have a life cycle where they are born, they mature, they perform a function, and they die. All living things go through that.

"A cancer cell is born, but it doesn't mature. If it's a breast cancer cell, it has forgotten how to become a normal breast cell. It remains youthful. The one thing it does remember is how to divide—more slowly than a normal cell.

"Young cells have the ability to reproduce. Mature cells can no longer reproduce. Because cancer cells don't mature they are forever youthful, and therefore they are eternally capable of reproducing. Also, because they don't mature they don't function and they have no commitment to die. They do die, but they live much longer than normal body cells."

I was beginning to think of these cells as little people—not that I was sorry to see the forever youthful cancer cells get knocked off, wasted, demolished by the big guns of chemotherapy. But big guns devastate large areas besides the target.

"We all know there are side effects of these chemotherapeutic agents. Please tell me about them."

Dr. Saiki's chair squeaked as he adjusted his position. Always a teacher, he spoke slowly and deliberately.

"The side effects can be divided into two major categories: side effects that relate to cell proliferation, and side effects that do not. Body systems that proliferate fairly rapidly are the blood, the lining of the mouth and the gastro-intestinal tract, the lining cells of the surface of the eye (the conjunctiva), hair follicles—all these are very sensitive to the side effects of chemotherapy.

"Those cells that reproduce more slowly are not a problem. Bone and muscle cells do not grow rapidly, so they do not suffer side effects—except if, through a separate mechanism, they are sensitive to a particular drug.

"Typically, this group of side effects includes hair loss, sores in the mouth, itching eyes, and things like that. Also suppression of your white cell count, making you susceptible to infection, and suppression of your platelets, making you susceptible to bleeding.

"The other group of side effects are not related to cellular proliferation. Those kinds of things are nausea, constipation; some patients have increased pigmentation of their skin. If you miss the vein and the drug invades normal tissue outside the vein, it can cause acute, severe, inflammation of the tissue."

Oh, how well I knew that scenario!

"There are other potentially damaging long term effects. The drug adriamycin can damage the heart, and that's long term. Once it's damaged, basically it's permanent. A small percentage of women of childbearing age become sterile with aggressive chemotherapy, and about 80% of young males will become sterile with certain kinds of chemotherapy. That's permanent too. There may be other side effects that we don't know of."

"More subtle?"

"Yes, more subtle. Children are being watched over years, just to see if there are things that we may not see early on, that may happen ten, fifteen, twenty or thirty years later."

Someone knocked on the door. In walked a young doctor with a puzzling case to discuss with Dr. Saiki. A woman's pathology report showed cancer cells almost to the margin of the breast that had been removed. Other complications made it difficult to decide upon a course of treatment. I tried to be politely unobtrusive in the background, but I was impressed with the fact that there were no hard and fast guidelines to follow. The patient's feelings and wishes were being honored as much as possible while the best course of therapy was worked out between these two physicians.

After he left, I commented on my observations. "There's certainly a lot of intuition involved in practicing medicine!"

Dr. Saiki smiled agreement. "Oh yeah ... oh yeah! In teaching, you have to teach the student how to think. Like...you know this is a Colorado columbine; How *do* you know it's a Colorado columbine? So you have to figure out how do you know it's a Colorado columbine? Then you teach a student how to learn this is a Colorado columbine, or a leukocyte or platelet."

"It's like Zen."

"And it's quite an effort."

How to learn reminded me of research, so I asked, "What is happening right now in breast cancer research?"

"I think there are two major areas of research. One is understanding the basic molecular biology of breast cancer to identify new approaches to treatment and new drugs. The other is looking at the immune system and trying to find ways to improve it.

"A transplanted kidney is recognized as an intruder by the immune system and destroyed by it if immuno-suppressant drugs are not administered. The malignant cancer cell is only a little bit different from a normal cell. Like the stealth bomber can fool the radar system if built just right, the malignant cell can fool the immune system. If there were a way to make it more recognizable, the immune system could then destroy it."

"Has the survival rate increased at all?" I ask this question, because there seems to be a discrepancy between reported statistics and the people I know.

He looked perplexed. "The studies by the National Cancer Institute show that there is really no change, and I don't know why. It's really funny. When I take care of an individual patient whose disease is aggressive and she is at a high risk of recurrence — where I know that many years ago this patient would have died if I had taken care of her then — now, with intensive treatment, she's not having a recurrence of her breast cancer.

"You know, when biostatisticians look at the overall cancers and say there's no change in mortality in the past thirty or forty years, well, that's not true, in a sense. Hodgkin's disease is now cured most of the time. Testicular malignancies are cured most of the time. I'm not certain if it's the numbers or what, but somehow you don't see that change in mortality, or the curability of cancers in general. I just don't know."

As I have mentioned, I hate statistics. I know we need them for something, but it seems to me they can be made to support any point of view. I repeated the observation made to Dr. McIver. "Statistics are based on something that has already happened, and not on the now time. Right now, we can't tell from statistics what has been happening in the last five years."

"Right. What's going on now we'll judge ten years from now."

"So we're a lag-step behind all the time. Perhaps that accounts for it."

He poked a hole in my theory. "Not entirely. Because if you look at twenty and fifteen and ten years ago in breast cancer, you would think that every ten years the survival rate would be better. There's been no change there. I really have no idea."

"Well then, maybe you can shed some light on why breast cancer is increasing so dramatically?"

"Our population is aging," he replied earnestly. "When you deal with the incidence of breast cancer, and other cancers, the older you get the greater the risk of developing it.

"The other thing is that there could be environmental factors. In some states, the breast cancer rate is actually decreasing, in some there is no change, and in some the rate is increasing. Overall, the incidence seems to be increasing, but we don't understand it. We know that eighty percent of all cancers are related to environmental factors."

"Eighty percent?" I was shocked.

"Eighty percent, yes. And we don't inherit cancer—we probably inherit the susceptibility, or the resistance. It's like a family with tuberculosis. Maybe the mother and one of the children have it, but the father and the other children don't get TB. Why? They have all been exposed. It likely means the ones who are well are more resistant. The same thing is probably true of cancer.

"If you look at the Black population in Africa, the incidence of colon and rectal cancer (which is the #1 cancer in the adult population in the United States) is very uncommon. Yet if you look at the Black population in this country, colon and rectal cancer is very high.

"Years ago in Japan, the incidence of breast cancer was very low. So they thought it had to be racial, or perhaps genetic. Then as they looked at some of the customs (breast feeding was very common among the Japanese) they thought perhaps breast feeding was protective. As more studies were done they found that no, breast feeding was not protective. So then they looked at genetics again. In Japanese-American women they discovered the incidence of breast cancer was rising to parallel the American rate. So obviously it's not racial, not genetic, and it's got to be environment. When populations migrate, they change their habits, and the incidence of their malignancies changes to the rate of the new country they adopt."

But why? I wondered. You can know it's environmental, but tracking down the causative factor in the environment seems an insurmountable task. Diet, lifestyle, stress, toxic chemicals, toxic air, pesticides, more— what a soup! How do you identify the culprit? I decided to move on.

"Dr. Saiki, what makes a person do well or not do well in dealing with cancer?"

His dark eyes laughed, for he knew I was probing his intuition, not asking for facts.

"There probably are a lot of answers. The most important, obviously, relates to the stage of the disease, the aggressiveness of the disease. If the stage is more advanced or the tumor more aggressive, the patients do not do as well. That's a critical factor, and that's how we determine how aggressive our treatment should be.

"And then I'm sure attitude has a big impact. I do not believe that the mood of a person, whether he or she is depressed or not, causes cancer. There is no way in my mind that this can occur. It's not like smoking cigarettes causing lung cancer. Your being depressed is not going to cause cancer. On the other hand, being depressed is going to affect how well you do. I mean when your spirits are down you are negative, you don't take care of yourself well, you don't brush your teeth, you don't comb your hair. You just neglect yourself.

"If you are not depressed and attack it in a positive way, you take good care of yourself. You eat better, everything is better and you will do better. I feel that is important in terms of how well a person does, but how much of a factor it is, I don't know. There have been some studies done that show it doesn't affect the outcome, but I don't agree with that."

I remembered he had talked previously about feeling out of control. "Dr. Saiki, once when I was here for a checkup you told me one of the biggest problems is the sense of loss of control when a woman finds out she has cancer. I can certainly agree with that. But then you said there is more control than one realizes. What did you mean?"

"I would say our Western civilization is controlling. That is, we control our environment. The Native American, no; he lives with his environment. But in our culture we control it. If we are cold, we make our environment warm. We heat it up. If we are hot, we cool it off. But when you have cancer you discover you can't control that—make it go away. The way I imagine some of my patients feel is as if they are in a big room, cornered, with a huge lion slowly coming towards them. What do you do? It would be gruesome. But the truth is there are things that you can do.

"One thought, and perhaps this is wishful thinking, is that maybe by being positive you can help your immune system. If you are stressed, you suppress your immune system. For example, people get fever blisters. Their virus starts growing and they get fever blisters. You get a cold, you get fever blisters. It's the same thing. So one would imagine that if you are not stressed you hold the virus in check—it can't grow. If you are really depressed and stressed your immune system can't hold the tumor in check. That is one possibility.

"Then I remember reading a book about visual imagery. There was a patient I had who was just as sick as could be in the hospital. She had acute leukemia and she was septic, and I'd talk to her about that—and the most amazing thing was that even though she was so bloody sick she was constantly imagining little soldiers in her blood attacking the bacteria; and her factory, the bone marrow, proliferating and developing new soldiers to fight the infection. What was impressive about that was she was always so positive, even though she was so sick. The quality of her life was ten thousand times better than another patient I remember who was just terribly depressed and stayed in bed. That woman was fatalistic and withdrawn. She wouldn't even read stories to her child, who desperately needed her attention.

"And then, people can eat well. Eat better, and it's bound to help the body and all the systems in the body. It's just like exercising is bound to help a patient with heart disease. And if they have a heart attack, that heart has to be in better condition because they had been exercising.

"Just the feeling that we can do something, like mental imagery, gives us a little bit of control. Suddenly we realize that we can do something, and that makes a person feel a lot more comfortable."

Our allotted hour was up, but because of the interruptions I didn't get a chance to ask Dr. Saiki all the questions I had prepared. He apologized sincerely, and we made a date for a follow-up interview.

The next time, as I was settling into that never-empty chair, I heard Dr. Saiki across the hall, talking to a patient who had been under his care about twenty years. She was sick with a lung infection, and his concern was evident. He was making arrangements to hospitalize her, and I knew that if I were in that position I would appreciate all his attention. So I offered to come back another time when things were less hectic. The offer was gratefully accepted. Very polite and caring, this man, as well as a darn good doctor.

We did get back together again another day, to continue the conversation. I asked him some more questions about his background and training.

"Dr. Saiki, I am interested to know what training you had when you were in school, in such areas as nutrition, psychology, alternative medicine, that sort of thing."

"In basic sciences our psychology was called psychobiology. In clinical sciences it was really rotations in psychiatry."

"In other words, you went into psychiatric hospitals and worked there?"

"Yes. We had very little that relates to normal psychology. Everything was abnormal. In terms of nutrition, we did have some lectures in nutrition and biochemistry. Most students, including myself, really had very little interest in nutrition. It seemed we had so much to learn about diseases and abnormalities that occur with diseases, that when it came to nutrition it seemed sort of like everyday life. We really didn't devote much time to it."

I smiled, knowing that nutrition is now in the forefront of research. "Now, I think there's a different attitude towards it!"

"It's totally different now, absolutely," he agreed. "And then, what did we have in terms of alternative medicine? Zero. Nothing."

I smiled again. How things change in a few years! "It just wasn't part of our tradition, then, in any way."

"Right," he agreed.

I moved into another area. "I know that you have support services for your patients here. What are they?"

"We do have a nutritionist available, based at the University of New Mexico Hospital. Generally I don't refer patients who only have cancer. If they are also diabetics, for instance, and want to learn more about a diabetic diet, I'll refer them. If a patient specifically asks me to visit the nutritionist, even though I think their nutrition is fine, then I will set up an appointment. If they have trouble eating, I'll set up an appointment. But if they are otherwise healthy I don't send them over for nutritional counseling.

"We also have a full time Ph.D. psychologist, who is available to all our patients. In addition, he has set up some group sessions with patients. The other services are basically medical services, with all the specialties."

The phone rang. He started to ignore it, but I indicated he should go ahead and answer. It gave me a moment to refer back to previous notes so I could get more information about tamoxifen. He had explained that estrogen is more a feminizing hormone and progesterone is more a masculinizing hormone. When he hung up, I resumed:

"In my case, I'm taking tamoxifen to block the estrogen, but my tumor did not have any receptors for estrogen. Would it be possible to use progesterone in that case as a protective drug?"

"It would be the same thing," he replied. "If estrogen receptors are present it means not only would tamoxifen help people but progesterone may have a greater likelihood of helping them too. No, just because your estrogen receptors are negative, it does not mean that progesterone would be better for you. The only reason that I use tamoxifen in patients whose receptors are negative is that, interestingly, there is evidence that it has activity aside from its estrogen-blocking function. At the molecular biology level, tamoxifen seems to inhibit breast cancer."

"And they don't really know why?"

"Not precisely. There are a number of different mechanisms that have been postulated. Clinical studies have shown that about ten percent of receptor-negative women respond to tamoxifen. There has also been some evidence that, used in an adjuvant situation, it can actually reduce the rate of recurrence. Not delay it, actually reduce it. That suggests that maybe it can play a role in helping cure a person."

"If I were a young woman," I ventured, "I would seriously think before ever signing up for the big clinical trials of tamoxifen that are going on right now. It has a lot of side effects. It certainly does reduce a person's interest in sex. It gives people hot flashes, depression, etc."

"Yes, I feel that would be a problem. The other thing is that medicine certainly doesn't have much experience giving tamoxifen for many years to a thirty-five year old, and what its long-term effects may be. We don't really know that."

I leapt at the opportunity to get on a philosophical level with this physician. "You were talking about things happening with tamoxifen on a cellular level. That's a kind of interesting area. It seems logical to me that everything happens on a cellular level—"

"In a way you can't see."

"—in a way we can't know, necessarily."

"Well," he offered, "all hormones in the body and all functions are basically at the cellular level. It's just that these cells are teamed up to—

(I moved my arm upwards)

"move an arm—

(I scratched my forehead.)

"—to scratch your forehead—

(I laughed.)

"—to laugh! So it's an amazingly complex system."

I laughed again. "Oh, totally!"

"But it all starts at the cell."

I am determinedly trying to steer this conversation into philosophical waters. "I think that what is happening now in quantum physics is shedding some light on the mechanics of how that happens—which I am sure is of great interest to you because of your work. It would be nice to know exactly why these things are functioning as they do—if we will ever know exactly."

"That's right. It's very interesting. Knowing a lot about a disease has nothing necessarily to do with being able to treat it. There are patients that have diseases we don't understand at all and we do cure them. Then there are other diseases that we know every last little detail, including the molecular abnormality, and we can't do anything about it. Like sickle cell anemia. We know a single amino acid substitution in the hemoglobin molecule causes the disease, but we can't change that right now. That's a disease we know inside and out, but we really can't treat it."

"And then there are others that you really don't quite understand," I questioned, "And you can treat them?"

"That's right, and cancer is one of them. For years, there have been certain tumors where we can give chemotherapy and the patient will be cured. We have no idea why."

I wasn't getting too far in moving Dr. Saiki into the philosophical, so I returned to the practical.

"Somebody told me once that all the chemotherapeutic chemicals you use are classified as carcinogens. Is that true?"

"I don't know whether all of them are, but in a sense they all may be because they all affect DNA. If you create abnormalities in DNA you can imagine that it could cause a defect that could result in the development of cancer."

"Have you seen any of this in the chemotherapeutic agents you use?"

"Oh, yes. In terms of breast cancer, I'm not aware of any occurrence of cancer due to standard adjuvant or more aggressive adjuvant chemotherapy. Certainly in my experience, I have never seen a patient develop another malignancy as a result.

"On the other hand, in Hodgkin's disease treated with aggressive combined radiotherapy and chemotherapy, there is a risk of developing leukemia. I've had one patient do that in all my years. A drug called alkeran has been associated with the development of leukemia too. Another name for that is melphalan. Another name for that is phenylalanine mustard."

"Mustard gas?" I was incredulous.

"Yes."

"You said all the chemo drugs affect the DNA."

"Yes, the major impact in killing a cell is either inhibiting the synthesis of DNA or preventing it from duplicating itself in cell division."

"Do these changes last?"

"No. Only during the drug exposure."

That brought up some of the things I wanted to ask him about my own experience. It seemed to me I was still dealing with the side effects of chemotherapy.

"You said that the muscles and bones don't have lasting difficulty because those cells reproduce more slowly, and so they are less vulnerable to chemotherapy. Yet while I was undergoing chemotherapy I had a lot of trouble with my muscles. They became tight, inelastic, and I became weak."

"Part of that is related more to inactivity," he rejoined. "When we give you the chemotherapy we make you so miserable you just don't do as much as you normally do. It's like putting your arm in a cast. A month later you take that cast off and the arm has shrunk. It's because tissues basically atrophy with disuse."

"Yes," I agreed, "and yet I specifically tried to keep moving, getting as much exercise as I could. I became very weak, though. I remember my husband would take me on big outings up to the mountains—I needed a nature fix—and we would walk a hundred yards at the most and I was pooped. Even my hands, the strength in my hands—"

"One of the drugs called vincristine, that you got, causes a neuropathy, and so it can make your muscles more weak, especially your leg muscles. And then it also causes numbness and tingling in your fingertips and toes. Decadron that we give, is a steroid to minimize nausea and vomiting. That actually causes your muscles to become weak. So those could have contributed too."

"OK, and then the other thing that I feel was a result of chemotherapy was an inability to absorb nutrients, because my digestive tract was affected."

He thought a moment, rubbing his chin. "That's possible. I don't know that it has ever been studied, but my gut reaction would be that it's very likely to have occurred, because the cells lining the GI tract that are very important in absorption clearly have to be affected by the chemotherapeutic agents. So their absorption is going to be less good."

"Another thing that I think sometimes can be a problem—I don't know if you have encountered it—is candida overgrowth because of the courses in antibiotics that are part of the therapy."

"Right. Yes. That can certainly occur. It tends not to be a big problem unless you are using large doses of antibiotics over prolonged periods of time. Or if the person's immune system is significantly depressed."

It was nearly time for me to go, so I tried to wrap it up. "Dr. Saiki, what would be your advice to women about breast cancer? What would you suggest to them?"

"For women who have just learned their diagnosis—well, there are a lot of little aspects of that. There are a lot of factors that go into making the decision about treatment. The best treatment for the disease may not be the best treatment for the patient.

"What I'm saying is, suppose we have a treatment that was absolutely curative ninety percent of the time. I tell the patient that is the treatment she must have. Perhaps the patient tells me she does not want that treatment, she feels she cannot tolerate it. If the physician insists, the result can be that the patient doesn't tolerate it and she quits and does not return. Then the patient is unhappy and the physician is unhappy.

"On the other hand, if the physician had treated that patient more gently and more conservatively, she would have had the disease under control. She would have felt well, it would not have interfered with her lifestyle, and she would have continued to function. Then the patient is happy and the physician is happy.

"And so the best treatment for the disease may not be the best treatment for the patient. There are a lot of factors that come into making a decision. If the disease is aggressive, then the treatment has to be aggressive. If the disease is not so aggressive and it's very early, then the treatment can be more gentle. And if the tumor itself is very small, less than one centimeter in diameter, the patient probably doesn't need adjuvant chemotherapy or hormonal therapy, and certainly the surgery can be a lot more limited.

"I also think it is always sort of good, if the patient doesn't know the doctor well, to get another opinion. Just to make sure that the original doctor hasn't overlooked something. It's not likely that something would be overlooked, but it is possible. The diagnosis could be wrong. It may not be cancer, although that isn't likely. But it's possible. I've had patients, not with breast cancer, but with certain kinds of lymphomas where they were thought to be malignant, and our pathologist says no, it's benign. And I remember one patient I had who was diagnosed as having an aggressive lung cancer and the pathologist looked at it and it was basically a benign tumor. So I think it's always important, if there's anything unusual about it, to get another opinion."

"As patients," I commented, "I think we hesitate to do that for fear of, I'm not too sure—of hurting somebody's feelings, I guess."

"Hurting the doctor's feelings? No, no! I think another good piece of advice, which fits along with the same thing, is the patient is the boss. The patient is in control, and they never need to be afraid of that.

"I advise the daughters of my patients that are concerned about developing breast cancer that if they have a lump in their breast that they think is a problem, and they see a doctor who tells them to wait a month—I tell them they must get another opinion. If the other surgeon says he agrees with the first doctor, then sit tight for a month. But if you know it's a problem, then you demand that it be biopsied. If you know in your own mind that the lump is a problem, then you take charge at that point. Sometimes something may look fairly innocent to a doctor, but in fact not be innocent at all."

"But we are scared that it might be, you see."

"No," he said firmly. "Whenever you are scared or you are worried, that means to me it's not a problem."

"Why do you say that?"

"Well, when you feel, like, a pain in your shoulder and you think 'My God, is that my breast cancer?' it really means that it's not cancer. When you have cancer that is causing pain in your shoulder, you don't just worry about it, you *know*. Likewise, in the old days before the sophisticated mammography technology that we have now, most breast cancers were picked up by the patients themselves. They found the lump. The truth is that when I have talked to those patients over the years, they knew what it was. They knew immediately what it was.

"But in terms of routine screening, if a young woman has a mother with breast cancer, I think it is appropriate to get a mammogram at the age of thirty-five, a routine, baseline mammogram. It will show what her normal breast looks like. Then later on, if there's a lump and the mammogram is done they will have a basis for comparison. Mammograms in pre-menopausal women are more difficult to evaluate because breast tissue is more dense. In post-menopausal women, there's a lot more fatty tissue, which gives you tremendous contrast. So you can see the breast tissue much more clearly. So mammograms are much more useful in post-menopausal women; much less useful in pre-menopausal women.

"In the age group between forty and fifty, a mammogram would be appropriate every couple of years. But very importantly, the woman herself should examine her breasts once a month, a week after the menstrual period. It's like learning to play tennis by playing tennis. The young woman will learn what her normal breasts feel like by feeling them. Over time she will know what normal and abnormal is."

"But doesn't it vary during the menstrual cycle?"

"Yes it does. That's why it's good to do it one week after the menstrual period."

"So one week after the menstrual period there should be no lumps?"

"Not necessarily, but the engorgement will go away, and it's easier to feel the breast."

Time was up. I thanked Dr. Saiki and left. Walking out into the parking lot I thought about all the things that had helped me through chemotherapy. Nutrition counseling and supplementation had sailed me through without losing any weight. Acupuncture had released muscle spasms and kept my energy going. And then the others had helped me see my true self and sort out the garbage.

I thought back to the first day when Ted and I entered the Cancer Center. Then, I was a victim. Now I was a survivor, committed to wellness, thanks to all my healers and my burgeoning awareness.

I thought about how I met those people, and the wonderful places they took me on my journey. Acupuncture was a field of flowers—a field of energy flowers I had not seen bloom before.

And the woman who nurtures these beautiful flowers, transplanting them into the garden of my life, knows how to direct their energy to heal. Let me tell you about Diane.

Exploring New Energy Fields

DIANE H. POLASKY

The Acupuncturist and Shamanic Healer

"Hi! I'm Diane!"

This is an acupuncturist? I was expecting a white-haired crone. This pretty, smiling face behind the desk didn't fit. Maybe she was the receptionist?

Momentarily nonplused, I looked at the business card Judy Asbury had given me earlier. It said Diane H. Polasky, so I figured "Hi! I'm Diane!" must be the Doctor of Oriental Medicine to whom I had been referred. Yes, she was young; that didn't mean she couldn't be a doctor. Part of the aging process is the fact that the older one gets, the younger other people look. In my head I am still thirty-five. A mystery!

Anyway, just like most of my adventures, this encounter with Diane was conceived at Mary Carroll Nelson's house. Mary exists in the center of a vast web of contacts. In my life she functions as the dream-spinning Native American Spider Woman, sending me scuttling off to outer limits of the web, down many exciting silvery paths of discovery.

A few months previously, Mary had suggested I contact a Washington D.C. area endocrinologist and internist, Dr. Leonard Wisneski. Dr. Wisneski had given a speech at our Layerists' symposium on Art and Healing in New Harmony, Indiana, at the precise time I was having my mastectomy. His presentation linked body/mind/spirit to disease. Mary thought he might have some helpful advice for me.

He did. He sent me a list of recommended reading, and suggested that I consider either transformational psychotherapy or acupuncture treatment by a traditional acupuncturist. Such a practitioner could be contacted, he wrote, by getting in touch with the Traditional Acupuncture Institute in Columbia, Maryland.

Once, shortly before his letter, while I was waiting for a blood test at the Cancer Center, a very healthy looking woman sitting in line was talking to another patient. "...my acupuncturist said..." she confided. I never actually heard what the acupuncturist said; but despite the rakish hat and scarf obviously hiding a head as bald as mine, this woman seemed so radiant and full of life that I figured something good must be happening. That impression, stored in my mental computer, emerged from memory when Dr. Wisneski wrote me.

I had already begun working with Dottee Mella, who fulfilled the role of transformational psychotherapist, so the idea of acupuncture got shelved...until that day at Mary's house when a group of Layerists had gathered to share art and ideas over tea and chocolate-covered peanuts.

Judy sat next to me. With loving concern she asked how my chemotherapy was going. "Have you tried acupuncture?" she asked.

"No, Dr. Wisneski suggested it, but I haven't followed through."

"Well, if you're interested, I can refer you to one of the best. I've been going to her for a long time, and I've been treated by quite a few others, so I know. She's wonderful! Furthermore, she appreciates artists and she collects art."

That sounded like a really good recommendation. Thanking Judy, I glanced at the card she handed me. Diane H. Polasky, it said, followed by a string of mysterious letters: M.A., O.M.D., L.Ac., Dipl.Ac.

Synchronicity strikes again! It doesn't take brain neurons much synapse-jumping to recognize the relationship of Polasky to Ploski; but a less obvious fact is that Diane and Cynthia are the same name as well! Goddess Diana, the huntress, is supposed to have been born on Mount Cynthus, on the island of Delos. From that birthplace, Cynthia emerged as a synonym for Diana.

Diane Polasky and Cynthia Ploski—too meaningful a connection to overlook!

OK, God. I guess I am supposed to see this woman! I called her office that very day.

Had I ever had acupuncture? the voice inquired.

No, I really didn't know much about it.

Would I like to see an explanatory video?

Sure! I would stop by the office and pick it up.

So that is how "Hi! I'm Diane!" came into my life.

That same evening Ted and I watched the video. It explained the theory behind acupuncture: that there is such a thing as "Chi," life-giving energy, which runs through the body on specific paths, or meridians. If energy pathways are blocked, those organs relating to impaired energy flow are not able to operate at peak performance. The body is out of balance. Stimulating energy flow by inserting needles at specific points on the meridians will bring the organs back into balance and restore their efficiency.

The information made sense, but graphic pictures of porcupine people, needles protruding from arms and legs, sort of upset my stomach. It's just a psychological thing about needles—I look at the ceiling rather than my arm when they draw blood. Many others undoubtedly do the same.

Therefore I arrived for my first appointment with Diane with a certain amount of trepidation. Betty Rice had volunteered to drive me. Welcome support! In my hand was the completed four page questionnaire Diane had given me. It was the strangest medical questionnaire I'd ever seen. It asked such questions as "Are you usually hot or cold?" or "Which is your favorite season of the year?" all of which seemed irrelevant. I had so much to learn!

The receptionist (who looked even younger than Diane) ushered me into a treatment room. She told me to undress and put on a seersucker cloth garment that velcroed in the front. Thus attired, I lay on the table, cradled my head on a pillow, pulled a cover over my legs, and checked out the unfamiliar surroundings.

How intriguing! The walls were decorated with posters of modestly nude Oriental men and women. Lines were running up and down their bodies, and spots on the lines had cryptic markings beside them. These men and women faced each other, or stood beside each other, in some sort of antiseptic, totally moral dance of relationship. One poster showed an ear, full of lines and spots. I remembered somebody had told me acupuncture on the ears helped people stop smoking. Why?

Near the posters were Native American artifacts, hinting at Diane's interests and abilities outside the boundaries of traditional acupuncture.

Very quickly, relaxation replaced trepidation. It felt really comfortable in that room. Not sterile and threatening, but rather peaceful and nurturing. Womb-like. A meditative state began to overcome me.

But lest I feel too comfortable, those familiar, damned, negative thoughts intruded. My personal nemesis, fear, crept into the room and played with my head. He reminded me where I was in my treatment journey—halfway through the chemo, weak, victimized, hairless, help-less, hopeless. I was in a valley. No, deeper. An abyss.

That pit was closing in when Diane entered. She clasped my hand between her two warm hands and smiled hello. Everything would be all right! I was undone. Mommy just kissed my boo-boo. The unspoken kindness and concern wiped me out. Tears leaked from the corner of my eyes onto the pillow as this woman, half my age, mothered me.

Mommy handed me a tissue, helped me sit up and gave me a hug. I snuffled. Then, settling into a chair with my chart, she became the doc-tor again.

"Well, now, Cynthia, let's go over this questionnaire."

For a half hour or more we talked about my answers. I learned a lit-tle about yin and yang, and how all that applied to me.

Yin is female energy: passive, moist, cool, the moon. Yang is male energy: active, dry, hot, the sun. For optimum health, they must be bal-anced.

When Diane was satisfied that she had a good handle on my phys-ical and emotional state, she had me lie down again and continued the diagnosis.

"You're feeling my pulse?" I am thinking it is racing pretty fast because of apprehension about those needles.

"Yes, all twelve of your pulses. Six on this wrist and six on the other."

"I thought I only had one!"

"Oh no," she laughed, "and they tell me all about your internal organs."

"No kidding?" This was a pretty strange idea. I was used to X-rays and blood tests, blood pressure cuffs and stethoscopes for that kind of information.

"No kidding. Pulses have different qualities, different intensities. The more skilled the practitioner is in reading pulses the better diag-nostician she is." Her fingers played a piano melody on my wrist. Soft and deep, quick and slow. She delivered an encore on the other wrist, then noted the results on my chart.

"Acupuncture needles are only as thick as a cat's whisker," she remarked, daubing alcohol in strategic spots on my feet, legs, hands and arms. "I tap them in through a little tube, so inserting them does not hurt."

I was glad to hear that, although pain isn't what really disturbs me about needles. It's more the idea of something sticking into my skin.

Nowadays, we also worry about getting the HIV virus from needles, so I asked her about that.

"Most practitioners, including myself, now use disposable needles. However, for my ecologically minded patients, I also offer two other options. The first option is that of reusable needles, which are autoclaved at 250 degrees for two thirty-minute periods after being soaked in germicide. The state requires twenty minutes at 250 degrees, so we exceed state standards.

"The last option is the purchase of your own packet of needles that we keep here and autoclave after each use. No other patient uses those needles."

I opted to use the regular needles. Diane turned on the tape recorder, filling the small room with soft, relaxing music.

"When I insert the needles, tell me if they are uncomfortable. A feeling of fullness or aching is OK. It's the Chi. Stinging is definitely not OK. It means I have to make an adjustment."

A tap, a simultaneous tiny prick, and the first needle was in.

"That didn't hurt at all!"

"Of course!" she chuckled. Up one leg the needles tap danced; up the arm on the same side. Probably about ten or twelve in all. One in my arm began to ache, so I told Diane about it.

"Go with it until I have the one on the other side in place," she said. "They talk to each other."

Talk to each other? But sure enough, when the corresponding needle on the other side was inserted, the aching subsided.

When all the needles were tapped in, she attached an herb called moxa (which is known as mugwort here in the West) to a couple of the needles in my feet and lit it with a disposable butane lighter.

"Heat augments the energizing effect of needles," she explained in answer to my raised eyebrows. "Acupuncture can be used to tonify or to sedate; build or disperse. Now, will you rest for a while?" A pat on my shoulder, a smile.

My head, already beginning to feel a little detached from a rapidly unwinding body, nodded agreement.

"Good." Her voice softened as she left the room, closing the door quietly behind her. "Have a pleasant journey."

There I was, needles on fire but relaxed. Imagine! Lulled by the music, I freely enjoyed the fragrance of burning moxa. Soon, little electrical charges began playing around different areas of my skin. Just little tickles. What was in that moxa smoke? I could feel the energy moving!

Wow! How interesting! As I lay there, beautiful colors of magenta, blue, green, purple, kaleidoscoped behind my closed eyelids. Slipping into that marvelous floating state between sleep and wakefulness, aware of feeling light and free, delicious shivers of energy coursed over my skin....

A quiet knock and Diane reentered.

"Time to come back now," she whispered. "I'm going to take the needles out."

"Already?" It had only seemed a few minutes.

Awareness, filtering back from that delightful place, wherever it was, found me on the table again, being divested of needles.

"Was it the moxa?" I mumbled, thinking it had indeed been a trip. A trip and a half!

"No, moxa doesn't do that—it was the needles." She smiled. "How do you feel?"

"Wonnn-derr-fulll..." my voice trailed. "Like I melted into the table...don't want to get up...."

"Have to bring you back," she laughed, feeling my pulses again. "Better." She reached for some more needles. "Turn your ankle in. A needle tapped in, and suddenly a mild electric shock made me jump.

"Sorry about that. I have to ground you, bring the energy back down." The other ankle got the same treatment, then both wrists. Again the pulses were consulted. "Much better. Take your time getting dressed. I'll see you in the office and give you some flowers."

Flowers? What did she mean? I slowly slid off the table, feeling light as air. Whose reflection was that in the mirror? It looked relaxed, younger, flushed, happy. Stepping into my clothes was easy. Muscle tension had disappeared. My body moved freely.

Diane was waiting for me at the reception desk. "Here, drink this. These are some Bach flower remedies from England that will help ground you and help you feel more centered."

She handed me a paper cup. I drank. It tasted fresh and fragrant. Flower essences! How lovely!

Betty was sitting there. "Glad your friend brought you," Diane remarked. "People don't realize how altered they can be, especially after the first couple of acupuncture sessions. It doesn't always happen, and it usually gets better with subsequent treatments, but that's why we give you the flowers and have you sit a while."

I slid happily into Betty's car, and into a restaurant for lunch. It felt like part of me was still hovering somewhere above my body. Betty just smiled and tolerated this euphoria like the good friend she is.

After lunch Betty and I attended a discussion group at (guess where?) Mary's house. More tea and chocolate covered peanuts—Mary's specialties—and other good stuff, including stimulating conversation.

To explain what happened next, I have to back up. A few months earlier, wrapping Christmas gifts, I realized my right hand was acting clumsy. Tying bows was impossible—the thumb just didn't work right. It didn't open up and it had no strength. That was my surgery side, so I thought perhaps it was what the Reach for Recovery woman had warned me about, tight arm muscles. But how could that be? I stretched my arm religiously! Then I considered it might be a result of chemotherapy. Actually, I never did figure out what caused the thumb to malfunction, but gradually it got worse. By the time I first saw Diane it was severely restricted.

So it was with great surprise and shock that sitting around the table at Mary's after my first acupuncture treatment I suddenly realized I could open my thumb with ease!

"You guys!" The group's conversation stopped mid-sentence. "My hand! I can open my hand! Look!" I flexed the hand open and closed like a door hinge and wiggled my thumb around, flapping the hand in circles like a bird in flight.

Marilyn and Ilena and Mary and Betty and Judy all must have thought I was crazy. I knew it had to be the result of the acupuncture session, so I told them all about my visit with Diane that morning. It felt like a miracle had happened.

I was hooked! The euphoria and muscle release lasted about twenty-four hours, but each time I went back it happened all over again. Bit by bit, the muscle release lasted longer and longer, and pretty soon I had complete use of the hand.

I visited Diane twice a week for the remainder of chemotherapy and during the radiation therapy that followed. To be honest, it was the only place I felt really safe. No white coats, no chemicals, no drugs, no mysterious, threatening machines, no fear of what might be wrong inside that body which had betrayed me—just warmth and tender care and good feelings. And those wonderful needles! Now they were my friends.

I was aware that acupuncture kept my energy level up, and it pretty obviously released muscle spasms, but I didn't realize how much it also benefited the immune system. After starting acupuncture, I never had another illness or infection, even though the chemo brought my white blood cell count below 1,000 every three weeks.

I still see Diane for acupuncture about once a week. Eventually I won't need it as often. However, I do believe it is so helpful that I will see her periodically, to keep in balance and deal with stress. I don't know if it works the same for everybody, but for me, it is wonderful!

That first time I met Diane, I could sense there was more to her healing ability than just skilled needle technique. It became obvious she operated on an intuitive as well as a technical level.

When our conversation led into other aspects of healing, Diane revealed that she is a practitioner of transcultural shamanic healing, as taught by Dr. Michael Harner. Harner is an anthropologist who studied shamanism with the Indians of Ecuador and Peru. He wrote a book entitled *The Way of the Shaman*. He also started the Foundation for Shamanic Studies, which conducts training workshops across the U.S.A. and abroad.

A shaman is a person who is able to enter other states of consciousness to find information on behalf of a client. Probably all of us can do this to some degree, but we do not recognize our ability. Certain people are trained to "journey" to other states of consciousness in a focused way, to help or heal those in need. This is known as shamanic healing.

There is nothing weird about other states of consciousness. They are familiar to us in the form of daydreams, night dreams or that lovely state between sleeping and waking. The exalted feelings you get from a special piece of music or from a church service are altered states of consciousness too. Being caught up in a good movie, a soap opera, a book... You get the point.

Two of the shamanic techniques Diane practices in addition to her acupuncture are called shamanic extraction and soul retrieval.

Long before being able to move to the Southwest I had become fascinated by Native American spirituality. From childhood I devoured the National Geographic that came every month. I remember sitting for long hours in mother's wingback chair, traveling back through those pages to the Incas, the Aztecs, the Egyptians, the Native Americans.

Cynthia, go play outside! You spend all day in that chair reading! The voice still echoes.

As an adult I read Frank Waters' *Way of the Hopi.* The ceremonies and beliefs felt curiously familiar. I yearned to be closer to that culture, eager to experience these techniques as an aspect of my healing. I trusted Diane—it seemed she would be a good person to introduce me to such mysteries.

So, eager to know more by moving deeper into that realm, I arrived at Diane's office one day in early spring to experience a shamanic extraction. I was not quite sure what it would produce, but I was open, ready for anything.

One of the treatment rooms had been cleared. A green blanket lay on the floor. Nearby was an assortment of paraphernalia: a rattle, a bird bone whistle, an abalone shell, a glass of water, a feather, a sage smudge stick.

Diane welcomed me with a hug, as always. "Take off your shoes and sit on the blanket," she instructed.

I settled down as comfortably as those chemo-stiff legs would permit, waiting for more direction.

"The concept of shamanic extraction is that oftentimes behind our illness is an intrusion, on a spiritual level, which takes up space in the body. Usually the intrusions (as we see them) are in the form of something commonly perceived to be ugly, like spiders, or snakes. They are not necessarily evil; they just don't belong inside of you. My power animals can be sent in to take the intrusions out. I only act as the 'visualizer' and facilitator. When the intrusions are extracted, the illness can be healed on a spiritual level."

"OK, so far. What do you want me to do?"

"Just lie down on the blanket. Leave room enough for me to lie beside you. Relax and let go."

I relaxed, closed my eyes, then opened them again as the scent of burning sage and cedar pleasured my nostrils. Diane was holding the smudge stick, waving the feather to direct the aromatic smoke at me, at herself, at the four directions, at heaven and earth.

"Cleanses and purifies," she explained.

I relaxed, enjoying the fragrance. It called forth mental images of mountains and mesas and clouds and trees and rivers of pure water flowing endlessly.

The ritual continued. Diane's singing, whistling, and rattling gradually lulled me into a magical feeling of lightness and anticipation. Anything seemed possible. Anything was OK, because I had confidence in this woman. I knew no harm could befall me, only healing. I wasn't worried, because Diane had told me she doesn't do the work, Spirit does. I'm for that!

Dim light filtering through the blinds illuminated sage smoke still lingering in the air, whirling slowly, dancing a vaporous pavanne. Fragrance sanctified the room. Quiet now, Diane lay down. I closed my eyes, just being there, sensitive to the woman next to me. Her breathing was deep and regular as if she were asleep.

Abruptly, she sat up, ran her hands lightly over my body, then dug briefly at my chest and belly, pulling something towards her.

Poof! Although my eyes were shut I knew that sound meant Diane was throwing whatever she had taken out of me into the nearest large body of water to neutralize it. More quick digging, then *poof!* again, several times. After the last breath she sat me up and, holding the crown of my head between both hands, blew several times into the top of my scalp.

Another hug, the ceremony was over. Back to ordinary reality, sitting on a green blanket.

"What happened?" I was impatient to know what she had found.

"There was a big spider web in your right chest, spreading down under your arm. It was charred, like it was burned, and several small spiders still clung to it."

"Yuk!"

"There's more. Near your liver was a kind of pipe, like a sink drain, clogged with green, moldy stuff, a small rattlesnake was coiled around your appendix, and there were "spores" of potential disease throughout your chest."

Even more yukky! I grimaced. "What did you do?"

"My power animals went in for me, and swept up the spider web. But there was still something beneath it, a big old tarantula, buried deep.

They dug it out, cleaned up the spores, cleansed the pipe and dispatched the rattlesnake. I threw them all into water to get rid of them."

"The intrusions won't come back?"

"They shouldn't—however when they were removed, there was an empty space inside of you. Since the universe hates a void, it could easily have been filled up again with another intrusion. To avert this, my power animals and I journeyed to find an animal who would help you by holding that space until you fill it up with something of your own. We found a big grizzly bear who volunteered to come live in your chest. And he says he just loves to eat bugs!"

"All right!" It felt good to have something fierce looking out for me on a spiritual level. "Does he have a name?"

"He said Na-tan. 'You must mean Nathan,' I told him. 'No,' he repeated, 'Na-tan'."

"Did he have anything to tell me?"

"Yes. He said you are doing the right thing with the herbs and nutrition and lifestyle. Not to change. But he said he had a message for you about death."

"Death?" A chill knifed up my back. "What did he say?"

"He said you must not laugh at death—neither must you fear it. You must make it your friend and travel the road of life together with it, or else you cannot be fully alive. You must not laugh at it, nor deny it, because death is worthy of respect. It must become your brother."

"Thank you, Na-tan," I murmured, sort of to myself. I was moved by the profound truth of his message.

Curiously enough, I have had "Bear Medicine," as the Native Americans say, ever since. In my own journeying into other states of awareness Na-tan Bear has been my companion. A rallying cry of "bear power!" helps me lift heavy objects or deal with difficult situations.

An Inuit sculpture of a laughing bear sits by my bedside, a silver bear adorns my necklace and Zuni bear fetishes hang from my ears.

Furthermore, in a statement of territorial possession, the only bear in 3500 acres of wilderness blessed our house site in Colorado by pooping on a special pile of rocks I had placed there in a sacred way.

I asked Teresa, my friend of Spanish ancestry, to come up with something appropriate to name the house, something delicate meaning "Place where the bear pooped." It took her a full day of juggling synonyms to come up with something that didn't sound crass, but the result is delightful. Purificación del Oso—a euphemism meaning "Purification of the Bear."

Anyway, to return to the extraction ceremony, Diane ended by having me drink a glass of pure water "to clean out the pipe" and share some cookies and apples that she laughingly claimed her "Jewish" Guides insisted she offer. "Eat, eat!" You might hear the same from Polish guides or German guides or Italian guides. "Eat! Enjoy!"

We did.

Before I left, Diane gave me a little red cloth containing tobacco and blue corn meal, with instructions to go out in nature and make a "thank you" offering. I drove out to the mesa behind our house and sprinkled the tobacco and corn meal around a juniper tree. In return, a gift for me fluttered on the branches of a tumbleweed—several bright yellow feathers caught in mid-flight by its thorny twigs.

Resting in the late afternoon, I mulled over the events of the morning. Stereotypes had been falling around me for months. The concept of a shamanic healer as an ancient medicine man in scary mask, chanting unintelligible syllables in a shrill voice and making threatening gestures with a spear, clearly did not relate to Diane.

She was none of that. She was a young, gentle, serious, attractive woman. When she spoke in ritual, no thunder was heard. When she shook her rattle, no lightning struck. Her voice was not shrill and powerful, but sweet and earnest. And yet, she believed so completely in what she was doing that I teetered past the edge of believing it too. One foot was in. I decided to stay open, because at that point in my journey I had come to truly know that anything is possible.

The weeks of chemo lumbered inexorably on. Regular twice-weekly acupuncture visits were obviously doing me a lot of good. Acupuncture doesn't grow hair back, but it relieves sore muscles and improves the flow of Chi, life force. Even though the chemotherapy was tearing my body (and the cancer) down, I really believe the acupuncture kept me functional, free from illness.

My unfolding faith in Diane's ability to summon the forces of Spirit to heal people was reinforced by the second shamanic ceremony she performed, soul retrieval. I stopped teetering near the edge and plunged right in.

Soul retrieval is based on the premise that certain traumatic events in a person's life cause fragments of his or her essence to flee in self protection. Their flight leaves a person's soul with missing parts, which must be restored in order to achieve completeness. The practitioner of shamanic healing can search other realms for these fugitive pieces and urge them to return and integrate.

This time as I lay on the green blanket I meditated while Diane journeyed beside me. It was the spring equinox, the day when the days and nights are of equal length. Balance; what we all would like to achieve. I thought briefly about balance.

Then my meditation moved in another direction, evoking some strong impressions. I visualized myself dancing. First I was a shaman, dancing like a Kachina in a white headdress with antlers and a white kilt. I had a strong impression of white. Then I saw myself as an eagle dancer with a white headdress and white wings, tipped with black.

Next the eagle dancing (myself) became a black bird, a raven, and I flew up high. Next, I became a snake, flowing down a waterfall. The impression was of flowing.

After that I became a brown, shaggy dancer. At first I thought I was a buffalo, but then realized I was a bear.

Diane's warm breath blowing into my heart and then my head brought me gently back to ordinary reality.

"Do you want to share your experience with me?" she asked.

"No, first tell me about your journey." The little skeptic inside me wanted to hear her side first, just to be sure my story didn't provide the inspiration for hers.

"All right. First I went to find if there were any animals who wanted to come with me to look for parts of you that were ready to return. Na-tan, your guardian bear was there, but no others. A spiderweb was the first scene that presented itself. There was a golden orb trapped in the center. I knew it was a part of your soul, from an incarnation previous to this one. It had been held captive by something or someone and had never entered this life with you.

"I approached and reasoned with it. I said you needed it to become complete. It agreed to come back with me because there was nothing to hold it back there any more. Na-tan wanted to carry it himself.

"Next I scanned for other parts of your essence that might be ready to return. I saw you as a newborn baby. Part of your soul left at birth because it knew there would be struggle in this life, and where it came from was so pleasant and happy. That place was Egypt, and that part of you was in the form of a black bird.

"I told the black bird that you had done the hard work already, and things would be more pleasant now—and you needed her. She agreed to come back, but insisted that you honor her by wearing a pair of gold earrings shaped like a bird. She showed them to me, so I could tell you what they look like."

I was beginning to be astonished at the similarities of impressions in my meditation to Diane's journey. "Confirmation" a small internal voice suggested. Where does that voice come from?

"After that, I saw you dressed like an ethereal being, in a beautiful white dress, like a wedding dress, very sad because you were going to lose your freedom. It wasn't exactly your freedom to do things, it was more your freedom to flow. I explained Cynthia has reached a point where she is learning to go with the flow of events, and that she needs you, as part of herself, to become whole.

"In her hands she held a sort of cylinder with a screw top on one end. She screwed another top on the other end, and very happily said she was now ready to come with me.

"The last vision I had was you at your first radiation treatment, with marks all over your chest. This part of you had left because you were afraid, very afraid, of both living and dying. I told her that Cynthia had decided to live, and to please come back because she was needed.

"She said she would, but you should get a pair of dancing shoes, because you should do a lot of dancing.

"When I blew these parts of your essence back into you, Na-tan wanted to keep the golden orb. He will keep it safe inside you."

Oh wow! The key words were all there. Bear, white, black bird, flow and dancing. But there was more.

"Diane, when I was born my mother crossed her legs and kept me back because she wanted to wait until the doctor got there."

Diane nodded wisely. "That might be the part of you that decided to not be born."

"And my mother has exactly such a cylinder as you described. It's an old fashioned perfume bottle that holds two different kinds of perfume. There's a barrier in the middle and a screw top on each end!"

She nodded again. "You still have work to do with your mother, Cynthia. She did not mean to cause you to struggle to be born, she just complied with other peoples' wishes."

That rang a bell. "I have always been too compliant, just like her. I've stuffed my anger and I've stuffed my power. Maybe that's part of why I got sick." An echo from Dottee again.

"Perhaps. Oh, by the way, your soul parts have a message for you. They said to be glad, because it is the beginning of a new life for you, and you will be well and happy."

I like messages like this from non-ordinary realities. They are useful affirmations. Hearing them, believing them, repeating them to yourself sets in motion positive energies.

On the way home I stopped in a store and found the earrings, just as Diane had described them, and in another store a pair of beaded moccasins, perfect for dancing.

Next day, writing in my journal about this experience, I thought about the symbolism that joined her vision to mine.

Symbols are powerful messengers. They are ideas sent and received on a sub-language level. In graduate school I learned that we cannot possibly process even a tiny bit of the information with which we are flooded each day, so we create symbols and stereotypes.

Just think of the symbols that are part of our everyday life—the cross or crucifix, the sun, moon and stars, apple pie, the flag of our country. White symbolizes purity, gold symbolizes worth. Most of what we experience is coded into symbolic forms. We don't notice them, for they are so much a part of our life. We just don't pay attention. Dreams use symbols and puns (which function as word symbols) to give us information.

Religion is full of symbols, some of them wildly mystical. For instance, did you ever ponder the Trinity, or Transubstantiation—the changing of bread and wine to Christ's body and blood? Literally! That's about as mystical as you can get—but don't forget saints and guardian angels. They are symbols too. Useful and comforting.

It is no surprise that so much of our spiritual awareness comes in the form of symbols. Keys (that symbolism again) to open doors to new understanding. Shamanic work is rich in symbolism. On a different level, so is acupuncture.

Flowers are beautiful symbols. Roses are love, violets are healing, daisies are sunshine, lilies are peacefulness, orchids are beauty and grace. The life energy that animates flowers is the same life energy—Chi, Prana or Mana—that enlivens—en-*live*-ns—us.

Acupuncture embodies those kinds of symbols. It is a field of flowers, blooming all at once, a riot of color, blending together to achieve harmony and balance.

All those letters after Diane's name can be translated as follows: Master of Arts, Doctor of Oriental Medicine, Licensed Acupuncturist and Diplomate in Acupuncture.

On the bright August morning of our interview, Diane and I had breakfast at seven o'clock in her office. She keeps long hours in order to be available to people with various work commitments.

First I asked about those credentials.

Diane's undergraduate studies were at the University of Michigan, where she earned a Bachelor's degree in Psychology as well as a Bachelor's degree in Eastern Philosophy and Religion. Her Master's degree is in Humanistic Psychology, from West Georgia College, near Atlanta. After moving to Washington, D.C., she attended massage school for two and a half years and was also trained in Bioenergetics and Feldenkreis.

While her former husband attended chiropractic school in Los Angeles, Diane studied acupuncture there for a year and a half, then dropped those studies when her daughter was born. Impressed with the training received during pregnancy, she became a certified instructor in the Bradley method of natural childbirth.

Later, after moving to New Mexico, Diane completed her acupuncture training in Santa Fe, at the school now known as the International Institute of Chinese Medicine, and under private tutelage. She went on to obtain her Doctorate in Oriental Medicine at Southwest Acupuncture College, also in Santa Fe.

As I surveyed her office that morning, I saw that Diane's surroundings are an extension of her many interests. The walls are decorated with original art from several of her clients. More artwork, Native American artifacts and paintings spill over into the reception area as well, where a large assortment of toys for kids and grownups are scattered. Yes, toys for grownups. Rain sticks, kaleidoscopes, rattles, more.

As we settled down with coffee and rolls, birds were still chirping reveille in a pine tree outside the door.

Pressing the record button on my little tape recorder, I began. "Diane, were you always a healer?"

She took a sip of coffee and replaced the mug. "Well, I won't go so far as to say that…but I've been led, ever since I was a kid. I remember starting back in sixth grade, carrying little notebooks around, writing down peoples' names and their problems."

"Little mother, eh?"

"I used to counsel them and take notes. So I guess it was appropriate that I went into psychology.

"It was after I received my Master's degree and started doing counseling work that I realized peoples' bodies held emotions as well as their minds. That's why I went to massage school, and started combining counseling with massage. Pretty soon as I was working on them I began to get visual images of the traumas people had experienced."

"You mean as you touched people, you saw the causes of their distress?"

"Yes. Working on the lower back of a woman who had been abused, for example, I would see what had happened to her."

"On what level was this occurring? Was it psychic interaction with people?"

"I don't know. I don't label things. But I started seeing visions through my fingertips.

"Then, as so often happens with people who go into healing professions, I got sick. Earlier, in graduate school, I had been told I would be in a wheelchair in ten years, because of my asthma. Back then, I could not even climb the stairs to my apartment.

"Later on, when I was in D.C., I was told I needed a hysterectomy. To go down the list briefly, there were bladder problems, ileocecal problems, hiatal hernia, fibroid tumors, endometriosis, and it just went on and on."

"You must have been a wreck," I sympathized.

She laughed. "Yes, and I was only twenty-five years old! I told the doctors I didn't want a hysterectomy. I was a newlywed, and I wanted a child at some point. My massage instructor at that time told me to go see his acupuncturist."

"And of course you did."

"Yes. I went to see her, and the work brought together everything that I had ever studied. It combined hands-on work, counseling, inter-action between people; and it had the spiritual/philosophical angles that were my training, that I lived with in my heart. It was like coming home! It was like everything in my life had been building up to this.

"Within a year after the treatments began, I went through a lot of positive changes. They couldn't palpate the fibroids anymore, my monthly cycles were back on track, I wasn't passing huge clots of blood like I had been.

"Oh, I forgot. I had hypoglycemia too, and after treatments my blood sugar balanced out. It was really a phenomenal experience. The healing and the growth I experienced under her care led me into acupuncture."

"That's when you began your training?"

"Yes, first informally in Washington, D.C. Then I started acupuncture school in Los Angeles and finished in Santa Fe. I've been in practice here in Albuquerque ever since."

"You certainly had a wealth of experience leading up to what you are doing now. Looking back, can you see how everything built towards a purpose?"

She nodded. "Right. They were stepping stones. And in the last few years the shamanic healing work I have learned through the Foundation for Shamanic Studies under Dr. Harner and Sandra Ingerman has been valuable. It has opened up a whole new realm. It has validated to me the fact that I have talked to Spirit since I was a little girl. It's a world I have always been part of, but I thought I was odd.

"As one person that I know puts it, 'In this day and age, if you talk to spirits, you hear voices, you see things that other people don't see, you would be put into a padded cell, or at least forced into intensive psy-chotherapy.'"

"Oh yes," I agreed.

"The more I do shamanic healing, the more I've seen it change my acupuncture practice. Now, when I take pulses and hold someone's hand to hear what their energy sounds like I travel in a very different way. I hear and see things very differently."

I scribbled a note to remember to mention that, in my own case, the shamanic work had been really helpful, augmenting the effectiveness of acupuncture and clearing away blockages.

"I can see that the two of them have combined in your practice," I affirmed. "You really can't separate them now."

Diane peered thoughtfully into her coffee mug as if it were a microcosm of the cosmos. "To me, working on the shamanic level is a way of seeing the world. It's a whole cosmology, it's a way of viewing life. I have a different vision now. It has changed my way of practicing acupuncture, but the acupuncture theories I follow are always the same."

I was glad she mentioned acupuncture theories, because it led to an area I wanted to explore. "Well, for the purpose of information, I'm going to separate the two for a while, and come back to the shamanic healing later," I said. "To explain acupuncture for people unfamiliar with it, please talk about its history and how it works."

"How it works," she smiled, placing her mug on the desk, "is a question that people have been trying to answer for thousands of years. Historically, it's anywhere from three thousand to five thousand years old. It originated in China.

"There are different stories concerning how acupuncture came about. Some of the books say during wartime, people were hit with arrows in certain places, and other places in their bodies would get better! But some of my more esoteric teachers would say—and which I now believe—that the Taoist priests, who were very spiritually advanced, were able to see energy on that level, and they developed acupuncture."

"So they could see, actually visualize the energy movement, and apply it to energy systems in the human body?"

"That's what they say," she chuckled. "I wasn't there! It makes sense to me, but Western medicine likes the arrow approach."

I finished up the last crumbs of the breakfast roll, wiped my lips with a napkin and tossed it into the wastebasket. Diane was marshalling her thoughts before diving into theory.

"Mind you," she said, "these are my own words. This is how I see it and how I have studied it. It basically works on the premise that the body is a bioelectrical unit; that we have energy flows moving through us that are affected by seasons, and by emotions.

"Chinese medicine doesn't differentiate between body, mind and spirit. They are all the same. What happens physically can affect the emotions. What happens on the emotional level as a child—I have seen this a lot—can set up propensities for energetic imbalances in certain organs later on in life.

"That's why it's real important to understand someone's history. I've seen it in body work as well. As a child you can't talk back. You are walking on the edges of what is happening in the family system, and the body says, 'I'll hold it for you.' On a cellular level, on a fascia level, on a muscle level, the body will hold those emotions. Chinese medicine recognizes that. They say there are seven causes of internal disease—imbalance in the seven major emotions."

This philosophy was saying in a different way what Dottee Mella had been telling me about burying your feelings. Chinese priests thousands of years ago were confirming what I was just beginning to understand about my breast cancer.

"Diane, what are those seven major emotions, according to the Chinese?"

"You must understand that it is the *imbalance* of these emotions that causes trouble. Everybody has these emotions. But lack or overabundance of any of them can throw off the organ systems.

"The major emotions are joy, anger, melancholy, grief, fear, fright and meditation. Meditation means over-thinking, thinking too much.

"Excessive fear, joy or fright can cause mental restlessness. Excessive anger can cause dysfunctions in the liver which can give rise to pain and distention in the rib area, irregular menses, mental depression, things like that."

I pressed her for more detail.

"It's a relationship," she continued, brushing a cloud of curly auburn hair away from her cheek. "Each organ system has a flavor, a color, a season, emotions, different body parts that it controls, different orifices that it controls. It's like a whole family unit. As the seasons change, specific organs come into play.

"There are different laws of relationship. One of them is called mother/child. For instance, if the mother doesn't make enough milk to feed the baby, the baby doesn't get enough nourishment, so the baby will cry. The baby shows the symptoms, but is there really something wrong with the baby? No! The problem is with the mom. Or if the grandmother is overly controlling and doesn't let the mother get enough rest to make milk to feed the baby, then the problem is with the grandma."

I remembered my daughter Melanie, who is a nurse, telling me there are more illnesses and deaths in the spring and the fall. Could this relate to Oriental medicine's awareness of seasonal influence? Now, all those strange queries in Diane's questionnaire were beginning to make more sense.

Diane was still talking. "There are seven major external causes of disease too, and imbalances in them can cause internal dysfunction. I'm talking about dryness, heat, summer heat or fire, dampness, wind, things like that.

"Just now, for example, late summer is 'spleen time,' and that has a lot to do with dampness. This is our rainy season. As practitioners we see a lot of joint pain related to dampness, respiratory problems, sinus infections, some cystitis. They are all disorders of the damp.

"In Chinese medicine, everything means something, and everything affects everything else."

"Sounds vastly complicated! Nothing seems to be excluded."

"Nothing. Nothing. Everything affects everything."

"Work, marriage partner, whatever?"

"Everything. We don't differentiate. Traditionally, Western medicine has been known to understand the physical systems that we have; the vascular pathways, the nervous system, things that you can see—"

"Things that you learn from dissection."

"—so in the beginning it was considered that acupuncture worked on the nerves. The gate theory, things like that about the nervous system. We said 'No, it has nothing to do with nerves. It affects the nervous system, but it has nothing to do with nerves.'

"It's based on the idea that, like a circuit board, we are bioelectrical units; that we have very specific pathways (the Chinese call them meridians) that run through the body. At various points on the body there are interconnections of these pathways where they have actually been able to determine that there's a difference in the resistance of the bioelectrical energy.

"These points are like a vortex, and the needles act like antennas. They affect the interchange of the energetic systems, bringing the systems back into balance.

"The whole concept of acupuncture and Oriental medicine is based on the idea of creating balance. When there is balance in the body, then the body/mind/spirit can heal. But you can only do that to the point where nature can be reversed. When we have gone too far out of balance, nature can no longer heal itself."

"Is that where intervention by Western medicine is helpful?"

"Yes, possibly. But it also can mean that death may ensue. Sometimes death is the cure."

I turned the cassette over and readjusted my position in the chair facing Diane's desk, while considering the relationship of Oriental and Western medicine. Everything I was learning pointed to their being able to work together for the ultimate good of the patient. Why don't they?

Each discipline has its unique advantages. Why should not these advantages be available to all, without discrimination? Isn't the well being of the patient more important than territorialism? Once the veil of ignorance or misinformation is swept aside, should not a new paradigm of cooperation emerge?

Putting those meanderings temporarily aside, I questioned Diane about the role of psychological introspection in acupuncture.

"These are my own views," she cautioned. "I tell my patients first of all that I don't 'fix' anything. I facilitate. I'm a traffic cop—I help direct energy.

"Acupuncture is like house cleaning. When you are dusting a house, you raise some dust in the air. When you are dredging the lake, you bring up the muck. We call it the Chinese box theory. Who you are in the present moment is like everything piled into a box, and you have to unpack the box.

"In order to create change, you must create movement. Acupuncture creates movement, which helps bring up stuff that needs to surface. If there are emotional fears and blockages in the way of healing, then they are going to surface. It's all part of becoming well again."

The tape recorder was misbehaving. I saw that the batteries were giving out, so I put some new ones in. Our fading voices picked up energy again. We were in business. My train of thought had switched to another rail, however, and we were back on the "how acupuncture works" track.

"We're moving in reverse," I said by way of explaining the switch, "to how you diagnose a patient."

"OK." She gazed off into space for a minute, then spoke quickly and firmly. "When a person walks in there are five basic assessment steps.

"The first one is *look*. We look at the person's 'shen' or spirit—their expression, the way they walked in, whether they look sad. We look for color in their faces to see if the cast is different from ordinary color. We look at their general appearance.

"Then we look at their tongue. In Chinese medicine tongue diagnosis is very important, because the tongue mirrors the body. Different coatings, different edge shapes, they all relate to something internally.

"The next is *listening*. You listen to any kind of body noises, and you listen to the patient talk. A groaning voice means one thing, whereas a sing-song voice means another. Some people don't talk, they shout. That's an indication as well. Different organ systems may be affected. There's a general overall pattern that we hear."

"I know my voice changes when I am under stress," I interjected. "I can hear it. It sounds strained and artificial, and it drives me nuts."

Diane smiled acknowledgment and touched the tip of her nose. "*Smelling* is another diagnostic tool. People have certain smells. For instance, if you have ever walked through a cancer ward you will be aware of a certain smell. Diabetics have a sort of sweet smell.

"Next is *asking questions*. I have a four-page history form that my patients fill out. Everything means something."

I remembered being introduced to that four page form. "I sure was puzzled by some of the questions."

"Everything means something in Chinese medicine," she reiterated. "For example, if you have pain, not only do we try to find out if it is stabbing or dull, or sharp, but is it better with heat or worse with heat?, that sort of thing. It all means something.

"And then we *feel the abdomen*. Abdominal diagnosis in Oriental medicine is different, and is very, very important. It also mirrors the body.

"After that we *take pulses*. There are six on each arm, and they correspond to different organ systems. Each pulse has approximately twenty-eight different qualities, but we usually only feel six to twelve of them. Some of them are very subtle. Some of the qualities we feel are fast or slow, full or empty, 'onion skin' or 'slippery.' "

"How delicate! It must take a long time to learn them."

Diane nodded vigorously. "Yes indeed. One of the teachers I met who had been doing this for fifty years could hug you, smell you, hold your hand, then tell you not only when you ate last, but what you ate, when you made love last, and on and on. He was just phenomenal.

"So this is how we make our diagnoses. We don't see illnesses as diseases, we see them as syndromes. A syndrome can manifest several diseases. For instance, you can have 'damp heat' in the lower abdomen. That can manifest as cystitis or fibroid tumors or menstrual cramps or pelvic inflammatory disease. Stagnation of liver Chi can cause tremendous numbers of problems.

"People ask, 'Can you treat my allergies?' We say we can treat you in terms of what your imbalances are. The allergies are a symptom of this syndrome picture. I don't treat disease. I treat people."

This was a totally different perspective on medicine from what I had been taught. "So you diagnose problems from the imbalances?"

"At least the basics. It's like layers of an onion. As you peel off one layer at a time you see how things change. We're not stagnant. We are always in motion. Motion is what life is all about."

"So what your imbalances are today might be different tomorrow?"

"Yes. It's the idea that energy systems are not fixed, either. You don't reach a perfect balance and stop. We move, just as the seasons move. As the seasons change, different energies come up. It's putting us in balance with the universe.

"Chinese people, 5,000 years ago, would come in for treatment at the change of seasons, at the equinoxes and solstices. They would come in on the anniversaries of their birth, or their moon cycles. They would come in when they were healthy in order to stay attuned to the changes around them. It's the idea of the microcosm and the macrocosm—they are one and the same. The idea was to keep them in harmony.

"Harmony fell away a long time ago, because as soon as we had electric lights, we started going to bed after dark. We didn't stay attuned. Modern technology reinforced our falling out of harmony."

"Are the energies that keep changing at the seasons the same as what you call 'Chi'?"

"There are many different names for Chi. Japanese call it 'Ki.' In India it's 'Prana.' Followers of Reich call it 'Orgone energy.'

"The Chinese have very specific kinds of Chi. You have Source Chi, Hereditary Chi; Chi that runs through your meridians, as well as Digestive Chi ..."

"What's Wei Chi?" Dr. Wisneski had mentioned it in his lecture.

"Wei Chi is basically what Western medicine would call the immune system," Diane responded. "Wei Chi is the protective defense energy of the body. It goes underneath the skin. If the Wei Chi is strong, imbalances in those seven exogenous factors like dampness won't go deeper inside the body. If your Wei Chi is strong, you may do battle, but you won't get sick."

"So increasing the Wei Chi..."

"Is like working on the immune system."

"So it's actual energy? Like electricity?"

"The Chi is simply energy."

"Cosmic energy?" I am trying to quantify this elusive substance.

"There's that kind of Chi too," Diane continued. "Every living thing has Chi. It's like essence. It's the essential energy of the body."

I quoted one of my favorite sayings, learned from a Navajo friend, Will Tsosie. "The Navajos have a saying 'Everything is alive and everything is in motion.' "

"Right!" Diane's eyes sparked with intensity. "And that's exactly the basis of Chinese medicine. The whole thing about Oriental medicine is that we keep the motion of the being in tune with the motion of the year and the universe. Treatment maintains movement."

"I don't think Western medicine recognizes Chi as that kind of a force. They seem to recognize a kind of life force that people either have a lot of or little of," I commented.

"They call it vitality. It's Chi too."

"It sounds to me like acupuncture is something that should be done on a continuous basis, like it was done 5,000 years ago."

"I call it 'tune-ups.' I send my patients post cards, usually winter and summer, to come in for tune-ups."

I checked my list of questions. "Is it true that needles can be used to increase energy or decrease it?"

"Yes, but different wording. Oftentimes you can tonify or you can sedate; you can build or you can disperse. There are different needle insertion techniques, directions of the needle, that will make a difference.

"We see it like a bell curve. You can monitor the length of time you need to leave the needles in by changes in the pulses. The pulses are incredible feedback. If you leave the needles in a certain length of time they will tonify. If you leave them in longer and go over the top of the bell curve, they will sedate."

"So the same needle will do both."

"Yes."

Next question on my list: "Diane, would you please tell me more about yin and yang? Yin is usually known as the feminine, right?"

"Right. Yang is more masculine. Yin is like water, it's coolness, it's downward direction. Yang is like fire, it's upwards direction. So anything that's quiet, dim, inside—as opposed to outward going, hot and bright—is yin.

"You can break everything down into yin and yang. Front and back, up and down. Take day and night, for instance. You have a yin part of the day and a yang part of the day. Take the yin part of the day and there's a yin and a yang part of that. It just keeps breaking down. They are basic theories. They are opposite, but they depend on each other. They support each other and they transform one into the other. If you get too much yin, then it becomes yang. If you get too much yang, then it becomes yin."

"It is a dance," I ventured, more than a little boggled by the complexity of their relationship.

"Yes, it is a dance." She extended the metaphor. "Everybody is doing the same dance, everybody is moving together. Like in the movies, when everybody is waltzing, it's just beautiful. If you have someone in there making the wrong moves, stepping on people's feet, you're going to get a chain reaction. As practitioners, we are going to teach you to dance better. That's how I see what we are doing."

Beautiful symbolism—movement, interplay, weaving together. This is medicine? Yes, but not in the Western modality. Healing, nonetheless.

My thoughts formed into words. "It's more than just putting people on a table and sticking them with needles. You create a healing environment. I know you use music, your own gentle approach, concern, good feelings. It's very important. I know that during my cancer therapy, your treatment room was the only place I felt 'safe.' I think this atmosphere is healing in itself."

"Everyone works a little differently," Diane said. "Some people follow a medical model. There are some who are excellent technicians. There are other practitioners who may not have as much training, but their treatments are phenomenal.

"For the past fifteen years I have been walking around with a Ph.D.

dissertation topic in my head, based on my own analysis and all the work I have done. My belief is that the relationship, the energetic exchange between patient and practitioner, is primary. The modality used is secondary."

"I think you'd find a lot of people agree with you," I seconded. "But unfortunately, a lot of people don't even consider using acupuncture as therapy because they think it will hurt."

"That's the question most often asked," she replied. "The only needles most people know are sewing needles, knitting needles, or hypodermic needles. They have this image of themselves laid out on a table impaled with hypodermics!

"I tell them they can fit four acupuncture needles into one hypodermic needle. They are about as thin as a hair, and there are different gauges and sizes, for different purposes.

"There are also ways to do acupuncture without using needles. We can use electricity, or heat herbs over certain acupuncture points. That's called moxibustion. Then there is cupping, which is suction work, and also acupressure. These are all specialized techniques that can be utilized in different ways. They will all affect the Chi."

"I found it very interesting, as you worked with me, to perceive needles relating to each other, 'talking' to each other, as you say. I could also feel different energy movement in my body, which is new awareness for me."

She nodded. "It's real important to know that the points we use aren't random. There are fourteen primary pathways in the body. Each has four or five secondary connecting points. You have a muscular pathway, you have what we call a tendino-muscular pathway, and you have got an internal pathway. There is an incredible network running through the body.

"Each of these meridians has several points of connection. Every organ system has an element. Take kidney, for instance. In Chinese medicine it corresponds to the element of water. On that kidney pathway you also have a wood point, a metal point, a fire point and an earth point. That is how the meridians all connect. It's like a whole family. The Chinese call it the law of five elements, and it's the pathway to affecting different organ systems than the ones you are directly working on. They are all talking, they are all dancing, they are all affecting each other. It is not random by any means."

I shook my head in amazement. "It's incredibly complex!"

"Now," I said as I moved further down the list, "when I was going through chemotherapy and radiation I came to you twice a week. What were you doing to help me?"

Diane rose, pacing briefly around the office, organizing her thoughts around my specific case. Returning to her seat, she leaned forward, speaking earnestly.

"The first thing I would say is that we were balancing what was thrown off by the chemo—also the shock to your system of learning you had this disease, and the emotions that go with it.

"Specifically, chemotherapy is very hot. I have found in other patients that chemo creates what we call a yin deficiency. There is a certain group of symptoms that we see in people on chemotherapy. We see hot flashes, loss of appetite, nausea, emotional restlessness, fatigue, insomnia, night sweats sometimes, restless dreams, general agitation and depression.

"We had to get rid of nausea right away, so you could eat and build up Chi. We also supported those organ systems that help metabolize food being taken in. We used points to keep the liver toned, because chemo is very hard on the liver system.

"I must clarify. We use words like liver, kidney and spleen, but it's not necessarily the physical organ we are talking about."

"Yes," I agreed, "that was a hard concept for me to grasp. Perhaps you could explain it for the readers of this book."

"Right. For instance, you have a physical liver. Everything goes through the liver, for detoxification. Chemotherapy—or any kind of drug—is hard on the liver. Usually it creates a deficiency.

"But also, the liver is the general of the body. It is the planner. It controls the smooth flow of Chi throughout the entire system. Emotions go to the liver first, according to Oriental medicine. So if your liver Chi is damaged, the Chinese see it playing a large part in the creation of hormone imbalances, allergy symptoms and more. The liver has to do with the element of wind in the body, affecting joints. You can have liver flaring up in the emotions—irritability, irascibility, anger."

"So when you say liver you are talking about the liver energy, in addition to the liver organ?"

"Exactly! The whole liver energetic system, not just the physical organ. When I talk to people about their livers, spleens, kidneys, it does not mean there's anything wrong with those organs."

"We think it does, because of our Western training."

"That was a lesson I learned as a student. An old woman misunderstood my teacher. She thought she was dying of liver cancer, but he was only talking about the liver energetic system.

"Another thing I learned as a student is to open doors for people gently, instead of kicking them open. We have a responsibility to assess the condition of patients, to see how emotionally fragile they are. We need to deal gently with them, respecting and honoring their space in the world.

"As an example, when a person comes in with chronic sinus and lung congestion, and I find out they drink three glasses of milk a day and eat cheese and yogurt and cold, raw vegetables, I don't jump all over them. I simply suggest they try cutting out the dairy, because it is mucous forming and clogs up spleen energy.

"Whatever you put in your body has special qualities. Herbs have different qualities, and affect people differently as well as foods."

"Herbs are an important aspect of Chinese medicine, aren't they? How do they work?"

"Everybody is an individual, and herbs work differently on different people. I have a problem with the mass marketing of herbs, which promotes the theory that certain herbs work the same across the board. How can an herb work the same for those people that seem kind of wet, full and soft like they are holding a little too much water, vs. these wiry, thin, hot-looking people?

"I'm not talking about the single, well-known herbs like echinacea, which has been studied and proven to boost the white count and improve immune function. I have a problem with the mass marketing of combinations of six or seven herbs. Putting specific herbs together to benefit individual people is a powerful way of healing.

"Some of the herbal work they are doing in China on immune disorders is phenomenal. It's starting to come to this country. Boosting the immune system through acupuncture and Chinese herbs is one of the areas people are really beginning to investigate. That's because in China they have done so much work on anti-virals, herbal anti-virals.

"Both Eastern and Western medicine have to work together for best results. In China they say if you have a tumor, you cut it out, and then use Chinese medicine to make sure it doesn't grow back."

"Exactly!" I agreed. "That's a logical approach."

"You have to use both," Diane agreed. I know that Oriental medicine and acupuncture have made a tremendous difference in people like yourself, going through chemotherapy. It helps keep the energy level up, the nausea down, the blood moving, the system stronger. The last thing we want is somebody on chemo getting a virus, when their immune system is weak.

"Hopefully as time goes on, Western medicine will see the logic of combining both approaches. It is beginning. I have been receiving referrals from doctors, mostly car accidents and personal injury cases, where the muscles are so traumatized that they can't tolerate massage or manipulation."

By now, we had talked so long that it was time for my own treatment. And we still hadn't even touched on shamanism! I didn't want to stop, so I opted to continue the interview, and to come back later that morning for my treatment. Diane took a break to return some phone messages, and I popped yet another tape in the recorder. I was thinking that although the interview was going into overtime, so much useful information was being presented that it would be a shame to cut it short. Besides, I was really enjoying the conversation.

Settling down in our chairs again, we focused on the way Diane utilized shamanic healing methods in her work. I wondered how she became involved.

"You moved into shamanic healing," I stated. "How did that happen?"

"I was very, very sick myself a few years ago. I went to a friend of mine who did shamanic healing work and underwent what is called a soul retrieval and extraction. At that point my life changed—it was like we got rid of things that were holding me back. It worked on me, re-empowering me. I was able then to see the dissonance in certain relationships in my life.

"It created a path for me, to the point where I was really driven to connect with the people who did this training. I went to every workshop that I was allowed to attend. They were conducted by Dr. Michael Harner's Foundation for Shamanic Studies, though I am sure there are other people who also do this type of training.

"I had been seeing a medicine teacher a couple times a year before that, and every time I saw him it seemed my life reflected positive changes. So I was prepared for the Harner workshops. They were a way for me to bring myself back to my own self and out of the illness. They moved my life in a whole new direction."

"So you went through the training courses, then started using what you had learned in your acupuncture practice?"

"Yes. In the Foundation's basic training program you learn how to journey. The whole idea is that in journeying you connect with spiritual teachers, or power animals, and start getting your own answers."

"I think we need to explain a couple of these terms," I interjected. "How would you define a journey? But first, how would you define a shaman?"

"I'm going to preface it by saying that a lot of this terminology and information can be clarified in Dr. Harner's book *The Way of the Shaman.* But to paraphrase him, a shaman is a person who enters an altered state of consciousness, traditionally by use of hallucinogenic substances (and more currently by drumming or other percussion sound) to make journeys into what are known as the Lower and Upper Worlds."

"I'll put that book in the resource section," I mentioned, writing a note on my yellow pad. "My understanding is that journeying is a way of moving into another, non-ordinary reality."

"Right. In my own words, it's based on the idea that using what they call sonic drive (drumming, or in some cultures singing or chanting) will create a shift in consciousness into non-ordinary reality."

"Sort of like a lucid dream state? Like I would imagine a dream state, but you are really there, instead of dreaming?"

"Sort of. Dr. Harner says it is safer than the dream state, because you will yourself to go there, and you can will yourself out of it. In dreaming you may not be able to extricate yourself from a frightening situation.

"I do want to say that it's not meant to imitate any Native American tribal thought. There are some people who are not real positive about this work, because they say we are white and this kind of thing hasn't been part of our culture.

"But I, and others, feel that we all come from heritages that have shamanic wisdom. Whether it's Old England, the Druids, the Norsemen, or in my case, the old Russians, everybody's heritage dates back to some tribal community. And every tribal community had some source of shamanic work."

I thought back along my family lineage, conjuring up visions of Saxons, Angles, and Franks running around the forests in masks and animal skins. Of course! "So it's everybody's heritage," I agreed.

"Yes, it's everybody's heritage. We all have these circles from which we evolved, and each of these circles had a form of shamanic work. This is one point on which Dr. Harner is real clear: not using any one tradition. He teaches what he calls 'core' shamanism. There is a basic core of teachings and beliefs, common to all shamanic practices.

"I want to preface what I am saying about the role of a shaman by stating that I don't call myself a shaman. I would never call myself that. I am a practitioner that does shamanic healing, but I will never advertise myself as a shaman. I have met shamans, and I honor them."

"It's like for years I called myself a painter, not an artist," I commented. "Can I call you a shamanic healer?"

She laughed, wrinkling her small nose. "You can call me lots of things, other things! But I'm just Diane, and I do what I'm told. The biggest, most gratifying experience in my whole life is that I am learning to listen to Spirit. I'm learning to listen to and trust and follow Spirit. And in doing that, I do healing work. I do shamanic work, but I'm not those titles."

"That's putting it in good perspective," I said. Diane is not one to be seduced by ego, as healers sometimes are.

"Anyway," she continued, "in shamanic communities there are certain categories of work the shaman does. One is divination, answering questions. Divination uses the movement of shifting into non-ordinary reality to seek out answers and find lost objects.

"Then there is shamanic healing. In shamanic healing spiritual intrusions are extracted. That is, something intrudes in the body (on a spiritual level, nothing physical) and the shamanic healer takes it out. It could be something that somebody could have zapped into you, or something that you just could have picked up, but it doesn't belong inside, nonetheless.

"Again," she went on, "knowing this all has to do with spirit, another category of shamanic work is called power animal retrieval. That is based on the idea a person can get sick from loss of power. There are certain symptoms—chronic depression, chronic illness, chronic bad luck, which can show up in ordinary reality.

"Power animal retrieval is based on the idea that the shamanic healer goes into an altered state and finds a spirit manifesting in animal form, with certain characteristics and qualities, that will come back to help the suffering individual. The shaman blows the animal spirit into the patient's head to help re-empower him or her."

I thought of my faithful spirit bear, Na-tan, and how I yell *"bear power!"* when faced with something really hard to do. It works. Of course if people hear me, they wonder. I've learned not to care about that.

"Then there is soul retrieval. This is based on the idea that at certain points in people's lives part of us runs away from traumas that occur. It's a survival mechanism."

This reminded me of the sexually abused children who do not remember anything about it until they are adults.

"Not every trauma results in soul loss," Diane went on, "yet sometimes soul loss comes from very simple things you would never suspect to be important. Going into an altered state and bringing back those pieces is part of the shamanic tradition."

In ways I perhaps never will fully understand, the soul retrieval ceremony had cleared away many emotional obstacles. I pressed her for more information.

"Some of the reasons for soul loss have been surprising to me. You can imagine the big ones—accidents, abuse, trauma; but I have recently become aware of more subtle ones. Sandra Ingerman, my teacher, says that alarm clocks can be a cause of soul loss."

"I can believe that," I laughed. "I hate them."

"One case I had last week was of the subtle variety. We went shamanically to this woman's bedroom. We saw her as a small child in bed having a nightmare, crying 'Mommy, mommy, mommy, mommy!' just terrified of being in that dark room. We saw her mother come in and tell her there was nothing to be afraid of, and to go back to sleep.

"It caused soul loss in that child. When her mother left, the child was thinking 'I have these feelings. I was just told these feelings didn't exist, but I *have* these feelings. But this authority figure said they are not real. But I *feel* this. If what I feel is not real, then I can't....'

"It set up this incredible dialectic through her life of not trusting her own feelings. It was something that simple, that moment of confusion.

"It doesn't happen the same way or at the same time for everyone, and not every person is going to experience soul loss. It depends on the individual. But it is amazing to me how it can occur, setting up a pattern for life."

"When you lose parts of your soul," I asked, "where do they go? Do they just go off in space?" I was intrigued by this shamanic paradigm to explain psychological patterns.

"We are going to reference Sandy's book *Soul Retrieval*, for that. I can't explain very well, but I'll try.

"I go to where the souls are. What I end up doing is sort of walking the person's time line, and—*poof!*—scenes pop up, and all of a sudden I move into a scene where there has been soul loss. Then I ask which parts are ready to come walk the person's time line with me back home. They come with me, and then I blow them back into the person's head and heart space. I have a feeling if you talk to ten people doing shamanic soul retrieval work they will have ten different things to tell you."

"Tell me more about shamanic work."

"All right. Another category of shamanic work is called psychopomp. It is helping people die, moving the soul from life into death, helping them make that journey. I've worked with that realm and the profundity of it is just awesome. You are helping the soul make that choice and get to the Light. Spirits are often trapped between this world and that as well, and need help."

I wondered if these trapped spirits were the ghosts we hear about— unhappy souls who don't even realize they are dead, yet have no home on this earth plane, or beyond either. The room was silent for a few moments, but it did not feel empty around us.

Diane leaned forward, tense with enthusiasm, her voice infused with awe.

"The strongest validation of shamanic work I ever had was a recent experience with psychopomp. A young man who was very spiritually conscious, was dying; he was between two worlds. The most amazing thing was that as we walked down the tunnel together in another reality, he would open his eyes in this reality and say things that would validate what we were seeing and hearing in the other world. So it was true. People in the room could hear it.

"As we were walking down the tunnel I was showing him the topography and where his path would go, and telling him about the people who would be meeting him. We were discussing it. He became very angry at one point, crossed his arms and sat down in the tunnel, and exclaimed 'I'm not doing this!' In ordinary reality he opened his eyes, looked at me and said *'goddammit!'* He brought that anger to this reality.

"I introduced him to his guide in the tunnel. He opened his eyes in this world and saw someone waiting for him that nobody else could see. He turned to me and said 'Who is that? You brought him, didn't you! That's my guide. That's for me!'

"I told him I did not bring the person. He said 'Yes you did. That's my guide!'

"He finally made his transition before morning. It was a good passing and a most powerful validation." She paused briefly. "I think people have a right to live fully and die whole."

I stirred in my chair, touched by the story. "I think our concept of death is changing very quickly as people begin to see it as transition. Birth must be terrifying too."

"Death is still a very scary issue," Diane replied. "I have seen people so afraid of dying that they are afraid to live! My experience as a childbirth instructor--"

"You help at both ends of it!" I interrupted, giggling.

"--is that both are profound changes." She remained serious. "I have found there is very little difference in coaching a conscious birth and coaching a conscious death. I see the stages of both, and the similarity is amazing. It says a lot about the sacredness of life.

"So this is all spiritual work," she summed up, "that has tremendous physical ramifications. It can create remarkable physical changes, but it's based on the idea of spiritual environments."

Our bodies reflect our mind and spirit. They are one. It's not a new theory.

At this moment in time I am listening to Diane telling me how physical healing is created through spiritual change. At this time as well, quantum physics is explaining the "why" and "how." Ancient cultures knew it worked, all along—long before sub-atomic physics was discovered.

"I want to say something for your readers about this altered state," Diane added. "In our training it comes from the sonic driving, percussion, dancing, that sort of thing. Many of the older cultures used mind-altering substances. Sometimes mushrooms or peyote or ayahuasca, depending on where a person lived. Ayahuasca is a root that is often-times used in South America to create altered states. Nowadays, we don't use those things. They are not necessary."

"So you use percussion," I confirmed. Anyone who has listened to music, especially loud, rhythmic music, will find himself feeling different. I remember when my son Jim was in high school, the kids used to go to dances and just stand around listening to loud, early rock music. I asked him what it did for him. He told me he liked it because the music went clear through him, brushing away all his cares and frustrations. There was no room for anything else but the sound.

Silence in the room brought me back from memories of Jim's high school days. I blinked my eyes and returned to Diane. "OK, so you do the shamanic healing outside of your acupuncture practice?"

"Right. I keep them separate. I don't usually even do it on the same day as I see patients for acupuncture. On the other hand, the more shamanic work I do in my life, the more it affects everything else in my life. Shamanic vision—it's a different way of seeing.

"Again, I want to be real clear that I myself do not do this work. Spirit does. Spirit---this can be a loaded word. It takes a lot of people off guard."

"Let's give it some synonyms," I suggested.

"Angels, guardians, guides, God, essential energy, masters, names like that. It's the God energy. I have always been real clear that Spirit does the work—to the point that if I get on an ego kick and think I'm doing something myself, something usually happens. Spirit lets me know.

"The whole point is that it's something bigger than me. It's something where I move outside of myself and Spirit works through me. It's not possession. We work hand in hand. I'm a facilitator between worlds.

"Everyone can journey. Everyone can learn to get their own answers from their own spiritual realm. I have an opportunity to listen well enough to learn how to walk between worlds. And so it affects everything that I do.

"When I take pulses now, the pulses are like drum beats. I sometimes journey while I'm holding a person's hand, feeling their pulses. I am hearing with my fingertips. It has given a sort of different twist to my acupuncture work, although I still treat patients in the very traditional Oriental way. It's just that my awareness has shifted."

This is what I sensed about Diane the first time she gave me acupuncture. She was hearing more than my pulses. It's a kind of communication that goes far beyond the norm; and I, as a patient, was glad she had that ability. I think she knew me better in a couple weeks than my parents ever did. By knowing me so well, she can treat me as a complete person, not the shell we all present to the outside world.

"If acupuncture's not a black and white area, shamanic work is definitely many shades of gray!" Diane continued. "The biggest thing—and this is something Dr. Harner said—is that it doesn't matter where the information comes from. What matters when you journey is the results."

"I'm glad you said that, because it brings up something I wanted to ask you. Sometimes it feels like this is all imagination. How does one differentiate between what is real and what is imagination? Or does one need to differentiate? I think you are telling me that it doesn't matter."

"It doesn't." She smiled at my confusion. "When I did an advanced two-week training with thirty-nine other people, we were journeying three or four times a day. We were seeing through rocks, we were talking to trees, we were doing some of the most amazing things. At one point we wondered if this was just mass psychosis! Were we just imagining? That's when Dr. Harner said it doesn't matter. We should not analyze it, trust it. There are certain guidelines you need to follow, but trust it.

"For me, validation has come from the fact that as I do this work with people, it is always right on the nose. It never fails. No doubt other people who have been in the field much longer have a thousand more experiences, but I have had enough in the last two years to know, and to trust. It is right on the money.

"In the beginning I used to worry what might happen if this, or if that—but Spirit does not fail. The whole thing about soul retrieval is empowerment. It's about becoming whole again, becoming re-empowered, regaining fullness, which is our right as human beings.

"Because," she added thoughtfully, "the more whole we are, our wholeness moves out into the rest of the planet, and the more whole and full the planet is. Spirit is more than cooperative. Spirit is more than willing to support our growth into fullness as human beings."

"Mmmm. That may be our eternal journey," I mused.

"Maybe," she added, "or our eternal opportunity. It's an incredible opportunity."

Shaking off the meditative pause following that profound statement, I moved on. "It seems like shamanism is spreading like wildfire. There are many teachers for ordinary people, in different contexts. Like there's Dr. Harner's system, the Huna paradigm, the Native American disciplines. Why do you think it's growing so fast at this particular point in time?"

"I think," she spoke slowly, the words flowing smoothly, like a river, "we are at a stage in our evolutionary development as individuals on the planet, that a lot of people are beginning to see things are much bigger than themselves.

"People are beginning to see we can't control things, and traditional religion does not have all the answers. Shamanism is based on the belief that everything is alive. I think more people are becoming aware of that."

Her voice rose, more intense now. "There is something bigger outside ourselves, and we are not alone. Everything interacts off of everything else.

"People are searching for meaning right now, at a time when they are not being given answers; or answers that hold enough meaning so that they feel full in their hearts.

"So I think it's part of the search, the idea that everything is alive, that everything is whole, that people are turning to things that are bigger than themselves because they feel a need to be a part of something.

"Our family structure has broken down. Our tribal units are non-existent. On a human level, people aren't relating to each other anymore as communities, tribes, as groups of people that can assist each other, and help each other survive.

"Shamanic work is one way of bringing people together more and helping each other heal. It's creating communities. It's one of the reasons that I have become a member of the clergy of something called the Circle of the Sacred Earth. It is a community that has a foundation in shamanism. The shamanic practices and principles are there. People have someone they can go to that will help give back to them spiritually, help them feel full and whole and powerful."

Diane's whole body seemed to emit soft energy. Words continued to pour out as if Spirit, not Diane, were forming them.

"I think it has been a question of cultural and social entropy, where people are feeling less and less empowered, feeling less and less whole, feeling less and less a part of things—and all of a sudden discovering that it's not true. And it doesn't have to be true. And you don't have to live like that anymore.

"So people are turning to each other, they are turning inside, they are turning to others who can help. Shamanism can help.

"In healing, there are obstacles. As a shamanic healer I look at a person and say "You are a whole person, and you've got these obstacles in front of you that are creating the problems in your life. I don't see you as *not* whole. I see you as *whole* and I see you as full, and these things that have occurred are creating a drag on that.

"We can do things to help you feel whole and full. I see you that way first. I don't see you as missing and screwed up and fragmented. I see your potential as being whole.

"...And that's how it works."

Her words hung in the air, as I closed my notebook and turned off the tape recorder. There seemed nothing to add. We sat in silence, transfixed by the moment, which was complete.

"That's perfect," I whispered.

That sunny August morning I left her office walking, as always, knee deep through a field of flowers...

...rose petals trailing from my fingertips...

...a crown of daisies encircling my hair.

Traveling On Light Rays

G E N E   W O N G

The Radiation Oncologist

We greet the rising sun with happiness when awakening every morning, for its light gives life to the earth, and life to us. Living without light is unthinkable; no, impossible. Even a few months without sunlight could bring our beloved planet to disaster. One of the theories for extinction of the dinosaurs is that the volcanoes erupted, spewed ash to block the sunlight; the plants could no longer create food and died. The dinosaurs, without food, died too.

Plants respond to light. Crocuses sense the lengthening day as their signal to push up through the snow. Morning glories glorify the morning, then shrivel away from night's velvet touch.

Animals respond to light. They are born, live, love and die in the seasons regulated by light. Shortening days tell the bear when to seek the shelter of his cave; the salmon senses when to struggle up that stream, spawn and expire.

Light animates us too, though we have lost much awareness of its effect upon our metabolism. We know that, flowing over our skin, it helps create the vital nutrient Vitamin D. We know our eyes admit it to our brains, and our glands respond. But there is much, much more we do not know and are only beginning to suspect.

Light is energy. Light is radiation. Light is illumination in every sense of the word. Light can destroy; light can heal.

The light is laser-like, hot, intense, penetrating and purifying the clear atmosphere of Arizona's desert. By summer, my journey to wellness was carrying me through just such a landscape; but it was the internal landscape of the UNM Cancer Center, and the intense concentration of light was for healing, like the Hindu Goddess Shiva, by destruction.

After Dr. Saiki had released me from chemotherapy the beginning of July, I had a couple of weeks off before starting radiation.

I needed it! The last chemo treatment had left me pretty weak. It's difficult to imagine what my physical state would have been without the support of all the other healers that had become part of my life. All through chemotherapy, I had been working with Dottee Mella and Diane Polasky, plus my nutritionist, shaman and naturopath. The Army, Navy, Coast Guard and Air Force, all together, could not have supplied more effective defenders.

According to Dottee, radiation had been no big deal; so it was with a remarkable lack of anxiety that I presented myself at the Cancer Center to meet my radiation oncologist, Dr. Wong.

Gene Wong's reputation for being personable is well founded. He bounced into the examining room, smiling broadly, shook hands and pulled up a chair directly in my face.

"How're you doing? I see Dr. Saiki has been taking good care of you! You look great!" Dr. Wong's almond eyes crinkled up as his famous smile widened towards his ears.

Visualize a person whose entire being seems to be one big smile. Who could resist him? Nothing about Dr. Wong seemed intimidating.

Even the radiotherapy program he outlined felt pretty happy compared to chemo. Twenty-five treatments, once a day, five days a week for five weeks. No sweat. Even when he mentioned possible side effects, they seemed no more threatening than a mild sunburn from a hedonistic day at the beach. After all, I had been surviving long-term radiation effects for decades.

Yes, I already knew about those long-term side effects—found out about them back in 1972, when an article about a certain Dr. DeGroot in Chicago caught my attention. He had been doing follow-up studies on people who had received radiation therapy for acne or enlarged thymus back in the 1940s. I was living near Chicago when the article was published; so remembering my teenage acne therapy, I made an appointment to see Dr. DeGroot, expecting to get a clean bill of health.

Surprise. He discovered a lump on my thyroid gland. Surprise yielded to panic. Was thyroid cancer to be the long term result of the radiation I had received? It often is, Dr. DeGroot told me. Surgery at the Mayo Clinic proved the tumor to be benign, but that illusion of safety, by which we insulate and comfort ourselves, was shattered. Once

Humpty Dumpty falls off the wall, the shell is cracked forever. No super glue can mend it.

Another side effect of that radiation treatment was the development of frequent small basal cell carcinomas—highly curable skin cancers—on my face. To control them I just see a dermatologist every year and he takes care of whatever pops up.

This is why Dr. Wong's warnings about the danger of long term effects of radiation did not worry me. I thought: *I survived it. I'm still here. Besides, what do I have to lose? If thirty years from now I develop another cancer I'll be thirty years ahead of where I am now, and grateful for all that time to be alive. I'll be nearly ninety years old!*

"They'll probably have a sure cure for cancer by that time!" I speculated out loud. "Let's go for it!"

He was still smiling, but serious. "OK, let's set you up for a simulation."

"What's a simulation?"

"This is where we make a plaster impression of your body in the proper position, so that you are in exactly that same place every time we do the therapy. Also, this is where we set up the fields."

"Fields?" No flowers this time, for sure.

"Fields are the areas we treat. We'll mark them on your chest with a sort of magic marker."

Simulation didn't sound particularly threatening, so when I showed up for my appointment I was relaxed. But when I left, a couple of hours later, I was on the verge of tears.

The plaster mold part was pretty interesting. It reminded me of a sculpture workshop. They set me up on a table and poured plaster underneath my upper body. As it sets, it gets warm, and that feels kind of good.

The hard part was that before they poured the plaster, they stuck a wooden handle above my head and had me hold onto it for what seemed forever, while the technician took X-rays, and consulted with Dr. Wong to ascertain that I was in exactly the proper position. This was the side of my recently healed surgery, the daily stretching side, the side that doesn't give without pain, the shoulder that pops out of joint when overextended. Hanging onto that handle for a couple hours was like medieval torture.

Each positioning and x-ray check lasted about twenty minutes, at the end of which my shoulder and arm were paralyzed. A compassionate attendant had to pry my hand off the wooden handle and lay the arm at my side, where it slowly pulsed back to life.

Precision absolutely must be achieved in radiation therapy. The beam must be positioned exactly, in terms of depth and breadth, to avoid damage to heart and lungs. So I was glad Dr. Wong was a perfectionist—it's just that I wished I had taken something beforehand to relieve the pain.

When he was satisfied with the position of my body, Dr. Wong instructed the technicians to go ahead with pouring plaster.

Oh good, I thought, *this is almost over!*

Not so. More X-rays to make sure the cast was perfectly formed to support my upper body in that same uncomfortable position, grasping that wretched handle, to be sure the fields were in perfect alignment. When finally released, I was shaking, angry and nearly crying. Simulation had sounded so easy!

Before I left the room, a therapist drew the fields on my chest with a special magenta marker. I looked like a distorted map of Arizona, New Mexico, Utah and Colorado. With a little of Wyoming thrown in.

"You better wear an old T-shirt to bed," the therapist said, "because you'll never get this stuff off your clothes." So on the way home Ted and I stopped at K-Mart and bought a half dozen white cotton T-shirts to live in for five weeks.

But the fact is that as time went on I found I could get rid of the stains by using one of those "stain stick" pre-laundering aids. Remember, nothing is ever written in stone!

As it turned out, simulation was the worst part of radiation therapy. The only painful thing from then on was sticking my arm into that unnatural position for a total of no more than twenty minutes each day, while they beamed short bursts of photons into my chest from different angles. Between bursts, I was able to put the arm down, so it was not as hurtful as before.

The photon beam used in radiotherapy is generated by a linear accelerator. Each time the beam is needed, the machine generates it by the effect of electricity on sub-atomic particles. There is no atomic radiation, no reservoir of atomic fuel. When the machine is off, no energy is emitted. There are other, different, radiation machines, such as the cobalt machine, but the University of New Mexico Cancer Center does not use them.

Delivering healing therapy to breast cancer necessitates irradiating several different areas. Since I had a modified radical mastectomy, the entire right half of my chest was treated, from part way up the neck to near the lower end of the rib cage. Precise calculations determine the beam's depth of penetration. In the shoulder and upper chest area, it must reach underneath the collar bone, where cancer cells may lurk in the lymph glands. The upper section of the lung usually suffers damage as a side effect. This part is considered more or less expendable, because it is only a small area of the lung.

Further down the chest, radiation was administered obliquely, from the side, so that penetration into the body was shallow. Otherwise, the heart and major portion of the lungs could have been irreversibly damaged.

What highly technical therapy! It requires the skills of not only the radiation oncologist; but also a radiation physicist, who makes sure the machines are working properly, delivering the proper amount of radiation; a radiation dosimetrist, who calculates the number of treatments and the length of each treatment; and the radiation therapy nurse, who provides nursing care and information about how to handle side effects. The actual therapy is administered by a radiation therapist, or technologist, who runs the equipment and makes sure the oncologist's instructions set up during simulation are carried out precisely.

If I had received my total dose of 4,600 rads (radiation absorbed dose) in one shot, I would have been fried. To avoid that, 200 rads were administered each day, five days a week. Healthy tissue, being less vulnerable, recovers between sessions, I was told; but cancer cells, more vulnerable, supposedly do not.

Anyway, first day of treatment, Ted and I were directed to a different waiting room in the Cancer Center, down the hall from chemotherapy.

We were sitting there, Ted reading a magazine and I meditating on the significance of Light Rays in religion and their effects on healing, when a young lady popped up in front of us with a Polaroid camera. She snapped two pictures, gave one to us and kept the other. "Why are you doing this?" I gulped, clutching my blouse.

"So we make sure we get the right person," she answered.

"Oh." What was there to say? It seemed impossible that with all this preparation, my chest marked like a map, they could mistake me for a foot or belly job, but I suppose the Cancer Center must take all possible precautions.

I was wearing an easy-off partially unbuttoned blouse with nothing underneath. The schedule was tight. I was planning to finish unbuttoning my blouse going into the treatment room.

The photo turned out to be pretty funny— Ted with his mouth open in surprise and me clutching at the buttons, looking (and feeling) somewhat invaded.

"Cynthia Ploski"— the nurse looked up from her clip board. I followed her compliantly into the treatment room, fumbling with the remaining buttons. Looking up, I nearly fainted. Dominating the room reared a giant, monster machine, poised over a table with my plaster form on it—a slobbering mechanical vampire ready to suck my life blood. Grabbing the arm of a chair helped steady me.

To understand that off-the-wall reaction, I must explain my irrational fear of huge machines. Some people suffer from claustrophobia, others fear heights. I'm scared of big machines. Perhaps it was the horror movies that fascinated us in our youth, or maybe my pregnant mother was frightened by a Model T Ford automobile. Who knows? Whatever the cause, giant machines seem to have a sinister, sub-human consciousness, and they make me very nervous. Boiler rooms terrify me, engine rooms on ships scare me out of my shoes. Excavation machines, jaws gobbling up rocks and earth, seem like menacing, uncontrollable mechanical animals feeding hungrily.

One time, just out of college, I was working on the thirty-second floor of a thirty-three story building in New York City. It was an early morning after a late date. In the elevator, I foggily pushed the thirty-third floor button by mistake. Walking out of the elevator door, turning right by habit, I ran smack into the machinery that made the elevator run! Huge, arm-like pistons lumbered up and down. Gigantic wheels whirred, sounding like a huge monster breathing. I panicked; fled back down the stairs panting, shaking.

Such a reaction is not logical, nor is it reasonable. But that's why, when I saw that linear accelerator in the treatment room, it was all I could do to walk over to the table and lie down on the plaster cast. The huge machine hulked patiently in the background while the therapist positioned and X-rayed me for the nth time to be sure I was perfectly aligned for treatment.

Then the machine slowly approached me, lowered its head directly over my chest, blinking a baleful red eye. The therapist adjusted some screens to shield all but the field being treated, then retreated to a glassed-in booth and turned on the machine. *Whirrr*— it built up force—then *buzzz*—it zapped me. I didn't feel a thing.

Quite a relief.

Since the radiation therapist seemed to have the monster well under control, I began to lose my anxiety. More changes in position, more X-rays, more *whirrr* and *buzzz*. Again from another angle, then a short *whirrr/buzzz* from below, like a punctuation mark, and I was through.

Ted was finishing an article on the Old West.

"Through already?"

"Piece of cake, yeah!" I didn't tell him about the red eye and my shaky gut. It seemed like a pretty childish thing to admit.

After that first treatment, the monster machine didn't scare me. I was able to relax and visualize light rays killing malignant cells, not just in my chest, but by some sort of osmosis everywhere in my body. I saw those rays as divine energy, healing, destroying what needed to be eliminated. A laminated Catholic prayer card showing Jesus with light streaming from his hands was a comforting image I reflected upon every day while waiting my turn for therapy.

The daily treatment became routine: Get up, shower, eat breakfast, drive twenty miles to the Cancer Center, unbutton, climb onto the couch, grab the handle, *whirrr/buzzz*, button up, walk around the grounds and up and down stairs to regain some muscle strength from chemo, drive home. Those cool morning walks around the shady grounds were a pleasure in the hot Albuquerque summer weather.

No side effects appeared, other than some fatigue, which an afternoon nap remedied. Dottee had recommended using clear aloe vera gel on the irradiated area after treatment each day. It must have helped, for there was no reddening of the skin until the next-to-last treatment, and even then it was just like a very mild sunburn.

Such a daily routine, punctuated by weekly blood tests and visits with Dr. Wong, left little time for other activities. The weekends were free, however, and one of them brought a remarkable experience.

Friends Kenna and Del from Wisconsin came to town and took me to Santa Fe. There, in a huge white tent the size of a football field, nestled among the hill country piñons, a plump, beautiful woman named Mata Amritanandamayi, dressed in a shimmering golden sari, sat welcoming with hugs and caresses all who approached her. Hundreds of people patiently waited in line for their turn to kneel before "Amachi" and receive her motherly love.

As I entered the tent, storing my shoes and purse on a rack, I was thinking how well I fit in. Except for the lack of vestments, my just-growing-in hair made me look like a Buddhist nun needing a head shave! All around were people in saris, in sandals and robes, silently meditating or just listening to exotic music emanating from Indian instruments. The sound came from a small group of devotees at the foot of Amachi's dais.

It was nearly noon when we arrived, and Amachi had been sitting there for hours without a break. After lunch, she resumed her position, dispensing love all afternoon. The evening was to have yet another ceremony. What amazing endurance!

At last it was my turn. As I knelt before this motherly young woman, my heart melted with emotion. The strange music pounded in my ears. I laid my head in her shining lap. Gently, she stroked my back, then lifted my face to hers, quietly murmuring words I could not understand. Even so, I knew what they meant, for feelings transcend barriers of language and culture. They were words of love and comfort. After a few moments she pushed me at arm's length, looked me full in the eyes and began to vigorously rub my barren chest. She *knew*, and she was giving me a healing! Another brief hug and I had to surrender my place to the next in line. Before I left, however, she smilingly pressed a Hershey's kiss and a small packet of sacred ashes into my hand.

My eyes swam with tears, but not from sorrow. My heart pulsed loudly, but not from fright. Wiggly-kneed, heavy with some sort of fulfillment, I sank to the floor in prayer and rejoicing.

Every year Mata Amritanandamayi travels from her ashram and orphanage in India across the United States and through Europe, doing exactly this: refueling people with the energy of motherly love. Divine Mother manifests in many ways. Amachi is certainly one of them.

I understand there are others doing similar work. The whole world must be in need of hugs!

Returning to radiation treatment the next day I still felt warm inside.

As the treatments marched by, winding down, new excitement was building up; my son Michael had a delightful excursion planned. He invited me to join him and his roommate, Todd, for a week on St. John in the Virgin Islands as soon as my therapy was through.

Dr. Wong was not enthusiastic about the strong sunshine there.

"You must wear a hat and a blouse with sleeves and a collar." He smiled as usual, but his eyes were serious.

"Even in swimming?"

"Yes, even in swimming. Well, perhaps not the hat! I have irradiated you as much as you can take, from half way up your neck to most way down your ribs, and onto your shoulder. You must protect it from the sun."

"Because it will burn easily?"

"Yes, but also because you increase the risk of developing other cancer further down the road."

OK, I could handle a shirt, even in swimming.

There is some variation of Murphy's Law that states, "As soon as something wonderful happens, you get a test." Shortly before I was scheduled to depart for the Virgin Islands, at a checkup with Dr. Wong, he spent a long time listening to my lungs. At last he looked at me, no smile this time, and said, "There's something going on in there. I want Dr. Saiki to listen too. Your lungs crackle like frying bacon."

Oh rats. I could see my vacation dream going up in a puff of smoke. Bacon smoke. Dr. Saiki confirmed the crackling sound, and they held a short conference.

"You can still go to the Virgin Islands, but I am putting you on prednisone for a few weeks." The verdict was in, and I was relieved. Prednisone seemed a small price to pay for paradise.

Prednisone made me feel like I had consumed ten cups of coffee, but the dosage was gradually reduced and that jittery reaction diminished. When I returned, my lungs were clear.

Although the usual bladder spasms before traveling kicked up, this time I just took some over-the-counter stuff that calms it down and boarded the plane. By this time I knew the pattern. Having learned that my bladder is a stress barometer, and that getting ready for a trip is particularly stressful for me, I now take cranberry capsules for a week before I go. That seems to take care of the problem. I knew I did not need antibiotics, but people who are experiencing bladder spasms for the first time should have a urine culture.

A week in the Virgin Islands turned out to be the ultimate doctor's prescription. My lungs adored the warm, moist salt air, my shaky legs grew stronger from hauling jugs of drinking water up flights of stairs to our little camp/cabin among the trees. The weather was wonderful, the company delightful. I learned to snorkel in the clear, warm water, filled with corals and tropical fish of every shimmering rainbow color.

At first Michael and Todd swam on each side of me, ready to rescue me if I got in trouble. But soon I was independent and able to be one with the ocean and the fish. Delight and relaxation and joy are great therapy.

When I saw Dr. Wong again on my return, I was able to report I had worn my shirt and hat like he told me. But now the shirt had indelible mango stains from juice dribbling down my chin and the hat was decorated with a "lei" of tropical flowers Michael made for me.

At last the doctors were through with me—except for regular checkups that will last a lifetime. Now began serious physical rehabilitation. Time to get on with living. Time to implement all the changes and understandings that had come to awareness during my journey, which was far from over.

CONVERSATION WITH DR. WONG

Gene Wong received his medical degree from the University of Hong Kong. His original intent was to become a pathologist, but he changed his major field to radiation oncology because he preferred patient contact.

Because his wife is Canadian, he emigrated to Canada, and finished his training at the Manitoba Cancer Treatment Center and Princess Margaret Hospital in Toronto. His fellowship was completed at McMaster University. A fellow of the Royal College of Physicians in Canada, Dr. Wong is certified in both Canada and the United States.

He came to Albuquerque as a result of a posting for the position in Canada. Feeling there was more career opportunity in the United States, he applied and was accepted.

As a member of the faculty of the University of New Mexico, Dr. Wong teaches, does research, some administrative duties, and patient care.

As I entered his tiny office for our interview I noticed how organized it was. But then, Wong is a perfectionist, for which I am grateful, so it is in keeping with his personality.

I wanted to know how radiation works. He smiled (of course) and clasped his hands together on his desk.

"Actually, I can't give you all the details, because it represents four or five years of training, but the essence of it is that radiation kills tumors by stopping the cancer cells from growing, or from reproducing."

"It interferes with reproduction?"

"Yes, it interferes with the division of cells. Now as you know, cancer cells kill patients by continuous growth. OK? So if we can stop the growth of cancer cells, or stop the division of cancer cells, then they will die, just because they have a limited life span. The use of radiation is to stop the cells from dividing, from so-called reproduction."

That was quite clear, but I wanted to know how it worked within the cell. "How does radiation interfere with cell division?" I asked.

"It is mainly through genetics. As you know, cell division is controlled by the genes."

"By the DNA?"

"The DNA, exactly. Radiation damages the DNA, or genes within the cell. Once the DNA is damaged, cells cannot divide normally. They run into problems during cell division that will abort the cycle. Then the cells just cannot divide."

"Doesn't this do the same thing to normal cells?"

"Certainly. It does not select only cancer cells. Radiation can affect both normal and cancer cells. The good news is that cancer cells are more easily damaged, because cells that are actively dividing are more sensitive to radiation.

"That's why, when we give patients treatment, they usually have problems with skin, with lining of the mouth or lining of the gullet, because these organs contain actively dividing cells. Cancer cells are the most active, compared to normal cells, because they are always dividing. So they are the most sensitive to radiation. And also, normal cells can heal, can repair.

"When we knock off a certain portion of normal cells, let's say in the skin or lining of the mouth or gullet, other cells can grow back. Just like after injury to your skin, you can actually see small islands of cells on new skin growing back. It's the same principle, because normal cells can be replaced."

"That sounds like good news indeed."

"Theoretically, yes. It is the reason we can give radiation. Because, as I have told you, number one is that cancer cells are more sensitive; number two is that normal cells can heal, can repair, whereas the cancer cells have very minimum potential to heal and repair."

I could not help thinking Dr. Wong's students are very lucky. It must be very easy to take notes, because he presents information so clearly. It was almost as if I were in class. I asked him my usual question about procedure.

"What are the steps you go through when a patient first comes to you?"

"I have to do a complete physical examination and history so as to know what the problem is. I then have to assess the approximate aggressiveness of the disease, and other medical conditions that might affect radiation.

"Sometimes you cannot give radiation to very ill patients, as they may have difficulty tolerating it if they are very, very sick. This is because, as I have told you, radiation depends partly on the healing of normal tissue. If the chance of healing is not good, we might have problems in giving radiation.

"The other things we look for include the location and possible spread of the disease. Of course, the location of the disease is very important, and whether it has spread or not. If so, where has it spread? Radiation is essentially a local treatment, as compared to chemotherapy. The chemotherapy drugs can circulate in the blood, whereas radiation affects a particular area only.

"So we have to be very precise in terms of deciding what area contains the tumor, and what area is at risk for harboring the tumor, even if there is not yet evidence of gross disease in that location. We will encompass all the potential area at risk.

"The other important thing is that we have to avoid treating vital organs, such as the brain, liver, kidneys, lungs and heart, if they are not at risk. If they do not contain tumor, we try to protect those organs as much as possible."

"You can be very specific in aiming the radiation, then," I commented.

"Yes, we can be very specific. There is new technology now with the use of the three-dimensional computerized plan."

"Tomography?" I guessed.

"Yes, tomography. Three-dimensional. That means you can really visually reconstruct the tumor and its relationship to different organs.

"Most of the X-rays or CAT scans will give you only a two dimensional image. But the latest technology enables us to create a three dimensional image on the screen, so we can plan the beam just to conform to the contour of the tumor. Tumor doesn't always come in spheres or rectangles, does it?"

That smile again. I shifted position in my chair facing his desk, mentally admiring the wonder of modern technological advances. How super that they are galloping ahead like knights in shining armor, to the assistance of all cancer victims.

I corralled those thoughts and brought them back to the room. "Dr. Wong, you do the planning of how you are going to treat the individual. You don't administer the radiation yourself, right?"

"Exactly. Now, after seeing the patient, after assessing where the tumor is, where to treat, that there is no contra-indication to treating the patient, then we will work first with the physicist. We will go through a simulation procedure, which you have gone through."

Oh, yeah ...

"Simulation means to simulate the actual treatment conditions," Dr. Wong continued smoothly, unaware of my inward groan.

"The reason for simulation is that we cannot see tumor from the outside. All we see is skin and some anatomical landmarks. But with the help of X-ray, CAT scan, MRI, we know the relation of the tumor to the surface anatomy. All we see of the patient is the surface anatomy. We cannot see through the patient and say "Aha!" I see your tumor inside of your abdomen."

"Not yet," I threw in, the galloping progress of technology still shadowing my mind.

"So we have to use a method to relate the image of the tumor from the X-ray, from the CAT scan, to surface anatomy. When we treat, the technologist has to follow some lines on the patient's surface, to direct the radiation beam. So that is the purpose of simulation."

"It sounds pretty mathematical."

"It is very technical, it's very mathematical. That's why we need to have a physicist and a dosimetrist. It's really team work.

"Now, after that simulation, we have related the location of the tumor to surface anatomy. Then we need to calculate how much dose of radiation to give through the skin so as to give a relatively higher amount to the tumor as compared to normal tissue. If you give more radiation to normal tissue than the tumor, that's not good." Another smile.

"After all the calculations by the physicist and the dosimetrist," he carried on, "then we know how much to give and all the technical details required to set up the patient so as to give the exact amount I want. The dose depends on the thickness of the patient and how deep the tumor is. That involves a lot of calculations, including computer planning. Sometimes we use multiple beams to fire at the tumor."

"At one time?"

"At one time, meaning of course in the same day. The reason for using multiple beams is to spare the normal tissue as much as possible."

I understood, then. Multiple beams means one after the other, from different positions. Not all together, but sequentially, during one therapy session, like they did to me.

"So after simulation you proceed with treatment. I know you do it a little bit every day for a specific amount of time to get a specific amount of rads. What is a rad, anyway?"

"The latest terminology now is to call it a centigray. One centigray is the same as one rad. It is the definition of a certain amount of energy. A centigray is a certain amount of energy absorbed by a certain amount of tissue through radiation."

"Do you always give a maximum amount in treating people? There is a maximum the body can tolerate, isn't there?"

"The amount that is given depends on the tumor, because different tumors need different dosages. Some tumors need a higher dosage to be controlled, whereas other tumors require less. One good example, as just a general statement, is lymphoma. Lymphoma, which is a disease of the lymph glands, usually requires less to be controlled. Cancers—carcinomas—usually need a much higher dose.

"So the first thing is the type of tumor. The second thing is the size of the tumor. If the tumor is only microscopic (microscopic means there is no gross disease), then usually we don't need to give that high of a dose. We need to give a moderate amount.

"But if there is gross tumor, visible tumor, palpable tumor, then we need to give a higher dose to give a better chance of control."

Dr. Wong leaned back in his chair and continued. "Now the other part of your question, what is the tolerant dose? In some situations, we know we can only give a certain amount of radiation.

"For example, let's say the tumor is in the brain. The brain can only tolerate a certain amount of radiation. Now we may want to give a little higher dose, but if we do that we may run a high risk of radiation side effects. In that situation we have to make a judgment; the possible benefit of giving more versus the risk of giving more. Different parts of the body have different tolerances."

As in all areas of medicine and healing, intuition is part of decision-making, I mused. Returning to the practical, I asked Dr. Wong, "What exactly is the source of the radiation?"

"In the good old days," he grinned at me, "we used cobalt or cesium. They are artificial radioactive substances made by a nuclear reactor. But now more and more we are using X-ray, artificially generated X-ray; generated by a linear accelerator."

"It's generated right there in the machine, isn't it?"

"Exactly. So the machine, you see, is the generator of the X-ray. When we switch it off, there is no radioactivity. But when we put current through it, the linear accelerator will generate high energy X-rays."

"I have heard the term photon used in relationship to the beam. How does that relate to X-ray?"

"When we talk about radiation, we are actually talking about different types of X-rays. Radiation is a very broad term.

"Photons apply to X-ray, which is one type of electromagnetic waves. Photons are part of the so-called quantum theory, which looks at electromagnetic waves as particles. But they are not particles, because they are light waves, just like sunlight. We see them as if they are particles, part of the light waves. It's really just a physics term for the energy in electromagnetic waves."

Quantum physics is way above me, although when I listen to Deepak Chopra or read Fritjof Capra's *Tao of Physics*, it seems to make a little sense. I can easily believe that inside every atom is a whole world of energy, identical with every other little world of energy, no matter whether it is in a rock or a human being. It helps explain why I have always liked rocks, nature, and animals. It helps me understand why I feel our oneness with everything, and each other, is a real, physical—though mysterious—fact.

We were on the shore of very deep waters, which I would have liked to plumb with him. But our time together was limited so I shifted gears, steering our conversation back to breast cancer.

"Dr. Wong, please tell me about the treatment of breast cancer."

He laughed. "Gee, I'm writing a chapter on the treatment of breast cancer, mainly for the radiation therapy technologist."

"Fantastic!"

"The treatment of breast cancer," he began slowly and deliberately, "is a combined modality. The first step is still surgery. Surgery is used to diagnose whether it is a cancer, or not. After the biopsy, if it is cancer, then the type of surgery depends upon whether we can preserve the breast, or whether the patient wants to preserve the breast.

"Nowadays people are more and more going for breast-conserving type of surgery. It doesn't mean it's better. It just means we try to preserve the organ as much as possible, without jeopardizing the chance of cure."

Another doctor who uses that "c" word— cure! I smiled to myself.

"It doesn't mean that it's a superior type of surgery as compared to mastectomy. It's about equivalent," he continued, unaware of my reaction to his choice of words. "It's about equivalent, if you choose your patients correctly. Hopefully, it can cause less psychological trauma to patients. But some patients prefer mastectomy, just because they don't want the anxiety of perhaps leaving some disease behind."

"Anxiety is a big thing," I offered, from my own memory.

"Yes. I have seen both ends of the spectrum. Some patients say 'No, I want to preserve the breast as much as possible,' even if they are not good candidates for conservative surgery. I have also seen patients who absolutely demand mastectomy because they know if they leave their breast behind they will worry about more biopsies all their lives."

"I have even heard of women having the other breast removed!" I added.

"Prophylactically, yes. It's at the other end of the spectrum. Surgery is certainly the first step, the mainstay of treatment. After surgery, we have to make a decision as to whether the patient needs more treatment. That means radiation and/or chemotherapy."

Dr. Wong leaned forward over the desk, tapping a pencil for emphasis. "The decision lies first in the aggressiveness of the tumor. We assess the stage of advancement of the tumor, the pathology of the tumor. We ask, 'Are there any lymph glands in the armpit involved? Is there any evidence to show that the skin is involved, or the lymphatics of the breast?' We have to consider all these questions, and then make a decision as to whether more treatment is necessary, to give the patient the optimum chance of controlling breast cancer."

"Who makes this decision?"

"It's actually a team effort. After the surgery we will talk to the pathologist and the surgeon, to make sure all the margins are clean. Clean means they do not see any cancer cells near the edge.

"We also need to assess the size of the tumor, the lymph nodes, etc., and talk to the surgeon as to what they see or what they think after surgery. The surgeon knows exactly the location of the tumor and if there is any risk of leaving tumor behind.

"In some cases, the pathologist will say, 'It's a clean margin.' But if the surgeon tells you, 'Hey, Gene, I have a little bit of concern over that part of the breast,' then I think you have to be a little more careful in interpreting the results. The surgeon knows best. He knows where he put his knife. If he is concerned, that might influence my decision whether to give radiation or not."

"So it's the surgeon, the pathologist, the radiologist and the medical oncologist ..."

"It's the four of us who make the decision."

"Then having decided, what radiation treatments do you use?"

"In patients who have conservative surgery, that is lumpectomy in which the surgeon just removes a small portion of the breast that contains the tumor, we usually will recommend radiation. The reason is that now we have very good data to show that in patients who underwent conservative surgery, there is an approximately forty percent chance the cancer will come back in the same breast. But if we give them radiation after the conservative surgery, then the chance of control will be improved up to ninety percent."

I was impressed. "The chance of control goes from sixty percent to ninety percent with radiation? That's amazing!"

"On the other hand, with patients who have had mastectomies, the entire breast removed, we will only irradiate patients who are at high risk of recurrent disease.

"Now you ask me, 'What's that group of patients?' That means they have positive margins or skin involvement, or the tumor is so big that we are really concerned there could be microscopic disease left behind, or lots of lymph glands are involved. Then we give radiation despite their having had the breast removed. But only in high risk patients. If they do not belong to the high risk group, then we usually do not give radiation after the mastectomy."

The telephone rang. Dr. Wong politely ignored it. I gestured to go ahead and pick it up. It gave me a few moments to change my tape recorder batteries and rearrange my note pad, realizing I was a member of that high-risk group.

He hung up the receiver. "Where were we? Oh yes, methods of treatment. The next question is, what about chemotherapy? The standard recommendation from the National Cancer Institute is that if the lymph glands contain metastatic disease, then the patient will need some sort of chemotherapy. It could be hormones or it could be chemotherapy.

"If the lymph glands do not contain tumor, that's a question. There is a lot of controversy regarding what we should do about this group of patients. My opinion is that we need to do further clinical trials to find out which sub-group of patients will benefit from the use of adjuvant chemotherapy if they have negative lymph glands. The bottom line is, it's very controversial."

I reiterated: "So then the purpose of radiation therapy for a person who has had a mastectomy is to irradiate the lymph nodes, to sterilize or to eliminate any disease in the area that is normally next to be affected?"

"If I understand your question correctly, you are asking when do we treat the lymphatics..."

"Well, in my case I know you treated the whole area. Why? Is that the general area of next contamination?"

"Yes. In your case we treated the chest wall, after removal of the breast. The reason is we would like to treat the original site that contains your breast. We feel that if there is any risk, the risk could be anywhere in the site of the original breast."

"Then the original breast extends farther than we think."

"Exactly! Now if you ask me, 'Can you be sure that you are including one hundred percent of the breast?' No, we cannot be sure of that because there are surgical reports that they sometimes find breast tissue over your scapula, over your abdomen---"

"Really! No joke?"

"No joke. This is real. But does it mean we have to treat half the body to cover every possibility? No. All we do is try to include the anatomical definition of the breast. Of course we know that some patients might have some breast tissue beyond that anatomical definition, because each individual is different. So is it worthwhile to over-treat ninety-nine patients just because of the possibility that one patient may have breast tissue in the abdomen or in the back? I don't think so.

"The risk of recurrent disease in that extra breast tissue is very small. The risk of cancer development of course is there, but it is very small, and we don't know which patient has that extra mammary tissue."

"That's fascinating," I blurted. "Do we have scattered bits of other organ tissue also?"

"Oh, yes, just like thyroid gland tissue could be anywhere. Most people would think a thyroid gland can only be in the neck. But that is not the case. We can find thyroid gland in the chest, inside the lung or what not."

"I had no idea!" I guess we are not anatomical textbook diagrams. We are more individual than we realize. *This gives new meaning to "His heart was in his throat" or "She has eyes in the back of her head,"* I thought to myself. My mind went off, searching for other comic examples. Dr. Wong looked at me inquiringly.

"Oh, yes." I stammered, coming back to the task at hand. "OK, I know that in my case you irradiated me at an angle—a tangent—for most of my chest, but the upper part you irradiated right through the lung. Why was that?"

"We would like to treat the breast but spare as much of the lung as possible. Your breast is directly over your muscle and chest wall. Underneath your chest wall is your lung, and we feel that the best way to treat the breast is to use two tangents so that we can include as much breast tissue as possible and spare the underlying lung.

"The reason that we have to treat your neck and armpit using a direct beam is to treat the lymphatics. Now the question of whether or not to treat the lymphatics depends again on the aggressiveness of the disease. It depends on the risk of harboring disease in the armpit and the neck after mastectomy. Again, the decision is individual.

"The way we treat the lymphatics is to put in a single, direct beam over the lower neck and the armpit. In that case, a certain portion of the lung has to be included. Technically, it's nearly impossible to use tangents to treat those lymphatics, so the only way to overcome the technical problem is to use a direct beam."

I stirred uncomfortably in my chair, remembering the frying bacon sound of my lung. The rest of my life I will sound like a barking seal when I cough or sneeze. Scar tissue, Melanie tells me. But I don't have any shortness of breath and I am able to utilize oxygen normally, so functionally the lung is still OK.

"That brings up side effects," I prompted.

"Yes. As I have said, radiation will affect both normal tissue and cancer tissue. And the more active the tissue, the more sensitive it is to radiation. Now, skin is a very active tissue, because you are replacing your skin continuously, although you are not aware of it. That is why skin is a very sensitive organ.

"Another side effect is radiation-induced inflammation in the breast. In some patients that causes engorgement, just like when you have lactation. The breast becomes full, distended, and could be tender because of the inflammation and increase of blood flow inside the breast. That's not a very common side effect, but these are the two most common side effects."

"What effect does it have on bone?"

"Part of your rib cage underneath the breast will be included, and that's necessary in order to treat the lymphatics deep in your breast. Radiation would not cause any direct damage to the bone, but it might cause fibrosis—scarring—in the bone and in the muscle. If the patient suffers significant trauma to the chest wall, that side of the chest will be weaker. But it doesn't mean it will fracture with normal activity. It would have to be a severe trauma. In that case it might fracture easier than the untreated side."

"How about the bone marrow?"

Dr. Wong thought a moment. "Ribs in adults have minimum bone marrow. It is mainly fat. So the effect on bone marrow should be minimal. Part of the collar bone and the humerus is treated, and in adults those bones also have minimal bone marrow."

"But does it kill off the bone marrow?" I was pushing the point, but he continued with his usual placid patience.

"Yes, it would affect some of the bone marrow, but we would not notice any significant suppression of bone marrow because the bulk of your marrow is outside that area."

"I know in bone marrow transplants they kill off all the bone marrow, and then inject new bone marrow, which will then grow."

"Yes," he chimed in, "because they rely on the new bone marrow cells to grow. If you knock off all the old bone marrow cells and don't give a transplant, then you cannot survive."

"I was just wondering if one's own body would do that, replace the marrow in ribs and scapula, from other bones that weren't irradiated."

"If it's radiation induced, then usually not, because that area will be scarred, and it will change the environment."

"I understand," I acknowledged. "Then the other way to get rid of bone marrow would be chemically, not with radiation, as chemotherapy would not change the environment."

"Exactly," he nodded. I think he was glad I finally got the point.

"But what about the immune system?" I asked, moving over a little in my line of questioning.

"Previously, way back," Dr. Wong stated thoughtfully, "people actually thought radiation could jeopardize patients with breast cancer. They said "Hey, you treat the lymphatics, you suppress their immunity, and that can cause flare-up of the cancer." That was in the '50s and '60s. But now, with more experience treating patients with chemotherapy and radiation there is absolutely no evidence to show that radiation jeopardizes the immunity and causes flare-ups of the breast cancer."

"I know there are long-term effects, Dr. Wong. I remember a paper I had to sign that said one possibility was that, years from now, another cancer could develop as a result of radiation."

"That's true. We know that radiation can induce a second, new cancer. But first we have to look at the risk of inducing a new cancer as opposed to the benefit of radiation. And remember, we are treating cancer, not a benign disease. So if you weigh between the benefit and the risk, we still feel the benefit outweighs the risk many, many times—"

"Perhaps by the time another cancer would develop, somebody will know how to cure the disease, anyway. Who knows?" I interrupted, hopefully.

"—and the risk is very small, one in several hundred," he finished.

"I understand the process of radiation creates toxins. Does the body just rid itself of the toxins, or are there things that can be done to help the body eliminate them?"

Dr. Wong raised his eyebrows in a puzzled expression. "From my point of view, we know that radiation can kill normal cells and cancer cells. Now, I don't know whether I would like to use the word 'toxins' because it would not create chemicals that are new to the body. Toxins, to me, are foreign to the body, do not belong to the body, and cause harm to the body. As far as I can tell, radiation itself doesn't cause new chemicals that are foreign to the body. Of course, there will be dead cells, there will be a change in metabolism in the body—but maybe that's what you mean by toxins."

"Yes. That's what I meant. Sorry."

"In that case, yes. Radiation kills cells, and can alter the metabolism of the region under treatment. It's a very complex process. The body just naturally gets rid of the dead cells."

I glanced at my watch, noticing how near the end of our allotted time we were. Dr. Wong had other commitments, so I moved into the question I ask everyone:

"What do you think causes cancer?"

"If I knew I would get the Nobel Prize!" he laughed. "In some cancers we know the risk factors. One good example is lung cancer. We know that smoking can give you ten times the risk of getting lung cancer. It's been proven over and over again through multiple epidemiological studies.

"In a lot of cancers, we do not know the cause. We know it has something to do with genetics. A good example is breast cancer. We know that if there is a strong family history of breast cancer, particularly in first relatives—mothers, sisters, first cousins, like that—then it puts one at a very high risk of developing breast cancer.

"Dietary factors may play a role, but again, it's a difficult thing to show and to prove.

"Hormones, contraceptive pills may be a possible cause of breast cancer—again, it's very controversial. My personal opinion is that I don't think there is any strong evidence right now to show that contraceptive pills increase the risk of breast cancer. There are numerous studies, but fifty percent of them show an increased risk and fifty percent of them do not. That's what I mean by absolutely confusing and controversial."

"How about estrogen replacement therapy?"

"Estrogen replacement is slightly different. If a person has a strong family history of breast cancer, certainly I would not suggest that person take estrogen, because breast cancer loves estrogen. It thrives with estrogen. So estrogen replacement could be a potential risk, particularly in people with a strong family history of breast cancer."

"That is why tamoxifen is being used now."

"Yes. There is a new clinical trial, a national one, to see if the prophylactic use of tamoxifen can prevent the occurrence of breast cancer. It's not for treatment, but for prevention in high-risk patients, in younger people with high risk factors."

"I would think the side effects of tamoxifen would make it quite difficult for younger women."

"Again, that's very controversial," he pointed out. "We know that tamoxifen has a potential risk of causing cancer of the uterus. That's one concern."

"It reduces a woman's interest in sex, too," I added, from my own experience. "And gives you hot flashes, dry skin and anxiety." Also from my own experience. Oh well, what drug does not have side effects?

"Dr. Wong, to wrap up, what advice would you give people about cancer?"

"My advice is simple—prevention is better than cure."

"How do we prevent it? The world of women, and some men, would like to know!"

His famous smile was rueful as Wong shook his head. "We don't know. First, most of the risk factors are beyond our control. You can't change your mother, you can't change your sister to minimize your risk. You are inborn with that risk already."

"Yes, but there is such a rise in incidence of breast cancer in non-risk people. I had no risk factors. And I understand that a great percentage of women developing it have no risk factors. Something else must be at work here too!"

"In breast cancer," he repeated, "the problem is that the strongest risk factor is still genetics. The other risk factors are so weak that we don't know if manipulating them can result in any significant reduction in breast cancer.

"One thing people have looked into is dietary fat. One theory is the more fat you eat the higher the risk of breast cancer. They looked into the diet of nurses, because they are easy to follow up and give good medical information. They tried to see if higher fat intake resulted in increased breast cancer, but the data is controversial. All I can tell you is that it is inconclusive."

"Has anyone looked at the Seventh Day Adventists as a group? For 100 years they have been vegetarians."

"Yes," he answered, "there is a study looking into that. They find the Adventists have the same incidence of breast cancer as everyone else. You can change your diet, but you can't change your genetics, nor your environment."

I am throwing out a pet theory now. "Dr. Wong, the world we live in has become increasingly loaded with toxins, pesticides, chemicals in our food in our air and water. Do you think this is a possible cause?"

"I would say yes, but can I prove it? It's very difficult, because from a scientific point of view you need so many patients. You need to design and control your studies so well that they are not influenced by other factors.

"If there are ten factors affecting breast cancer it is very difficult to control the other nine factors. If you cannot control those other nine factors, then you cannot make any conclusive deduction, saying that 'A-ha! Insecticide or herbicide is the cause.' There are too many confounding factors."

"So what do you recommend people do for prevention?"

Dr. Wong thought a moment, then looked at me earnestly. "For prevention, I recommend what the American Cancer Society recommends. Mammograms are important, no doubt. Many trials have shown that mammograms are very important in early detection. That's slightly different from prevention.

"Mammograms do not prevent breast cancer; they pick up early cancer, and we know that early cancer is controllable. Early detection is very important."

"Prevention, then, is really just leading a good life?" I queried. "Not smoking, eating, drinking in excess?"

"I can't see any harm in avoiding those risk factors, even if they have not been proven," he replied. "But it comes to quality of life. If people have been smoking for fifteen years and quitting affects their quality of life, then it's difficult to judge. But in my opinion, if something can reduce the risk and can be done easily, why not do it?"

"I realize our time is up, Dr. Wong," I acknowledged, "but please, just a couple more short questions?"

"Of course," he answered politely.

"Do you see any effect of mental attitude or emotions on cancer's cause or outcome?"

"Yes, certainly you have to look at the physical aspect and the mental aspect. Cancer is a big word. A lot of people are avoiding doctors because they are afraid to be told they have cancer. They are delaying or procrastinating just because of denial, simple denial.

"Denial has nothing to do with education, mental or socio-economic status. I have seen so many well educated people, including physicians, who deny disease. So yes, I think it is important to look at both the physical aspect and the psychological aspect of cancer patients."

"How about their mental attitude about their disease?" I pursued. "Does that affect the treatment or the outcome?"

Dr. Wong rubbed the back of his head and looked up at the ceiling before answering carefully.

"From a scientific point of view it is very difficult for me to prove that with a positive attitude you can have a better chance. It is nearly impossible to prove. But in many instances we know that patients who have a positive attitude can tolerate treatment better. If they can tolerate treatment better, then they will do better."

I thanked him, telling him how much I appreciated his clarity of thought and willingness to share his limited time with me; then gathered up my paraphernalia, exchanged smiles with him, shook his hand, and left the small office. *What a nice man,* I thought, for the hundredth time.

Walking out through the Cancer Center halls, I looked into the crowded waiting rooms. It was obvious that cancer does not discriminate. Small, bald children, mothers, ashen-faced men in wheelchairs, young women of child-bearing years, male executives, gentle old folk supported by their children and grandchildren—every age and race. It reminded me of another, earlier time at the Cancer Center, when I decided I needed to write this book.

That time was when I heard one in three people will have cancer in their lifetime.

One in three! That means statistically that for every father, mother and child, one of them will contract cancer. A third of our population! That's an appalling statistic.

So what are we to do? What power do we have to fight this aggressive disease? Medical science is forging ahead, with dedicated staff, constantly improving technology, and new drugs; yet it is barely keeping up with the surge.

There are other therapies—holistic, alternative therapies—that help people to affect the course of their disease. Perhaps if these alternative therapies are accepted by Western medicine as supplemental and effective, the statistics may improve. Shouldn't that be desired by everyone?

I was aware of those other therapies, because I found some of them on my healing journey. I also knew there are many more outside of my personal experience. They all center around that old/new concept that mind and spirit are inseparable from body.

By the time I reached my car in the parking lot I had decided it was essential that I include in the book information about these other methods of healing. I felt I should share my personal awareness, born of the belief that the dysfunctions of our bodies (our expression of self in this world) are reflections of dysfunctions in our minds and spirits.

Rooting out and exorcising those emotional and spiritual dysfunctions is what so many alternative healing therapies are about. Some, like acupuncture, massage and nutrition, deal with the body on a physical and energetic level. Others, like shamanism and transformational psychotherapy, probe the mysteries of those other parts of our being: spirit and mind.

I knew there are other realms of our existence. The Bible told me so. So did intuition, dreams, journeys, imagination, art, music, drama, love and psychic awareness.

That introspective drive home from Dr. Wong's interview at the Cancer Center reminded me once again of my hypothetical journey from Los Angeles to Albuquerque. By now, I decided, I had about reached the Navajo reservation—and as I continued east through the Indian country of my healing journey, I attuned my spirit with the Great Spirit that enlivens us all, asking that I might understand the deeper recesses of my soul.

Once again, a teacher came to me when needed. This time it was in the unlikely shamanic form of Alton Christensen, a white man, no feathers, no masks, just an extraordinary person with an extraordinary gift of journeying to worlds here, above and below.

I was ready to explore that path.

Visiting Other Worlds
Above & Below

ALTON   CHRISTENSEN

The Shaman

The first time I met Alton Christensen, I almost spent the night with him.

But that's getting ahead of my story.

I had just been into chemo long enough for my hair to fall out when (who else but my Spider Woman, dream spinner) Mary Carroll Nelson said to me, "Cynthia, I think you need to see Alton Christensen." Mary had consulted him once, and was impressed enough to include him in a book she has written about very special people, called *Artists of the Spirit*, under his shamanic name, "He Who Sleeps at the Foot of the Horse."

A shaman? Me? See a shaman? This was before Diane journeyed for me, so the idea was new, unheard of, and unquestionably on the wild side.

I come from a family and a culture that is terrified of anything unseen. They call it "occult" and make it a satanic word. As a child I was not allowed to play with ouija boards, or talk about ghosts, or visit fortune tellers or discuss extra sensory perception, *déjà vu* or anything pertaining to that shadowy world. Such close encounters with Spirit were shunned by disapproving frowns, averted glances—and feeling tones of fear.

I thought a shaman had mysterious, mystical powers, far above what we mere mortals possessed. As time went on, I came to understand we all have these powers, but for the most part they are not utilized. Shamans certainly do possess heightened mystical powers, but those abilities have emerged through the birth canal of personal suffering, soul searching, practice, surrender and trust.

Certain people may have a special calling to shamanism, just as certain people are called to nursing or ministry or theatre or art. But if they do not recognize their vocation, they may receive a wake-up jolt of no mean proportions.

Thinking I might be stepping off the deep end (but what the hey!) I nervously dialed Alton's number to make an appointment. First, he told me, I must see a woman in Santa Fe who is an astrological counselor and herbalist, who has successfully treated thousands of cancer patients through diet and herbs.

So one bright early December afternoon, Betty Rice drove me to Santa Fe to see her.

She turned out to be a comfortable, healthy-looking woman of early middle age, with a sandy pony tail and Bierkenstock sandals. I was expecting no more than an astrological consultation, but the discussion only partly dealt with those astrological forces contributing to development of my cancer. Most of the interview consisted of her protocol for treating it.

She told me that on the physical plane, cancer is a metabolic disease, caused by the improper digestion and utilization of nutrients. If we do not have proper digestive juices and enzymes, and if we flood our systems with indigestible foods, foods which are not right for our metabolic body types, we create toxins which harm us. So to cure cancer, we must change our diet so as to promote proper digestion and elimination. That way we are creating an environment where healthy cells can put malignant ones out of their misery.

According to my astrological chart, I have a tendency to give nurturing to others, but not myself. Dottee had said pretty much the same thing earlier. Yes, this creates resentment, another form of anger, and I guess I turned it inward. I was working on that already.

I was told I was not using my Mars energy. It rang a bell, from one other astrological reading, many years ago. At that time I had been urged to cut, slash and burn in making art—but the most Mars I could manage was gently tearing rice papers to put in my collages. I was not using that aggressive energy, male energy, yang energy.

She psychically saw me as a nun or religious person in many lifetimes, never having to deal with the problem of taking care of my own needs. I never learned how.

And she told me I am a healer. Dottee had said that too. It felt strangely uncomfortable.

The diet she recommended consisted mainly of grains and vegetables. Warming spices were good to use, to help promote digestion—but meat, most dairy and most fats were out. Her diet closely follows Auyervedic principles, so I bought an Auyervedic cookbook she had for sale.

I left that office with an armful of literature and a bunch of herbs. Those she felt would be most healing for me were pau d'arco, echinacea, yellow dock, red clover, milk thistle and combinations of herbs reputed to be blood cleansers.

Several of the compounds contained chaparral, which is one of the ingredients of Jason Winters Tea. Rather, chaparral *was* one of the ingredients of Jason Winters Tea. As I mentioned earlier, the FDA took chaparral off the market recently because a few (I heard it was four) people developed liver problems by taking too much of it. It may be only coincidence that a drug company came out with a cream containing chaparral to treat pre-cancerous skin lesions at the very same time the FDA issued its edict.

I personally know a woman who developed kidney failure from too much ibuprofen. (Advil, Nuprin, etc.) Warnings are currently being issued about the danger of taking too much Tylenol. Yet the FDA has not taken them off the market.

Putting this in the perspective of FDA-approved chemotherapeutic agents, big gun steroids and other highly dangerous drugs with severe or potentially fatal side effects, it makes me wonder just how much right we really have to treat our own bodies with natural herbs.

One of the other controversies that came to my attention was a conflict between holistic and allopathic medicine. To the holistic healer, cutting, poisoning, and burning are no way to heal the body. To the traditional Western healer, holistic approaches are at best ineffectual and at worst, quackery.

It was out of the question at that point for me to choose between the two. It was impossible to imagine not continuing chemotherapy and radiation, simply trusting diet and herbs to cure me. And, as Alton was to point out to me later, the journey through duality is to embrace the opposites, thus to walk through them—not to choose one or the other.

I didn't understand that then, but I wanted to hedge my bets, hitting the cancer from all sides. I was beginning to realize the relationship of emotion to healing. So despite warnings of what chemotherapy would **do** to me, I decided to follow through with it and supplement my healing process holistically.

It was a wise choice. As time goes on I hear a mellowing of the bellowing from both sides. Thank goodness, there is a movement towards combining modalities.

There exists an American Association of Holistic Physicians, whose members incorporate alternative therapies into their allopathic practices. Many physicians will quietly lay on hands or work with body energies. Nurses, especially, use healing energetics in their contact with patients in very individual and intuitive ways. They don't say much about it.

My dream would be a clinic staffed with a full array of medical doctors; and also chiropractors, nutritionists, transpersonal psychotherapists, naturopaths, herbalists, massage therapists, etc. That would really be a healing center!

But to come back to my story—fortified with information and herbs, I was ready to see Dr. Alton Christensen.

Our appointment was for the day of the winter solstice. Winter solstice is when the sun rises at its southernmost point. From this time on, days get longer. Dark begins to surrender to light. It is a potent symbol of emergence from the darkness of cold and fear into the warmth of enlightenment. How appropriate! I was in a dark mood as I drove, by myself this time, through falling snowflakes towards Alton's little home tucked away in the hills of Tesuque, north of Santa Fe.

I had left Albuquerque for Tesuque despite Ted's protests about the weather, fully intending to keep this appointment. Adding to the darkness was a gnawing sense of guilt about visiting a shaman. Maybe I only imbued Ted's grumpiness at my departure with disapproval. Perhaps he really did think I was out of my mind. Or it might have just been the threatening weather. (Probably the ghostly disfavor of generations of parents and ancestors hovered in the background as well. Who knows?)

Whatever the cause, guilt evolved into low-key anger and dogged determination. Anger, properly used, creates wondrous energy. There is nothing so exhilarating as righteous wrath! Especially for a person to whom anger is ordinarily denied. But in this case, guilt kept peeking around anger's corner, creating a certain empty ache in the pit of my stomach.

Snow started coming down more thickly through dull gray skies as

I guided my old four-wheel drive, four-cylinder Subaru station wagon north on I-25. By the time I reached Santa Fe, it was an incipient blizzard.

Confidently pushing on, I followed my directions to the fire station in Tesuque. Stopping at the bottom of Alton's driveway next to the fire house, I surveyed the situation.

The dirt road up to his home was a steep hill. The left side of the drive dropped off sharply to the valley far, very far, below. On the right beckoned a four-feet-deep ditch. About eight inches of snow blanketed everything.

OK, car, you can do it! Just use that four wheel drive. Remember all the snow in Chicago, and the snowy hills in Vermont? Stick it in low, get a running start, and don't stop for anything until you get to the top! OK? Go!

Holding my breath, gripping the steering wheel, squinting through the snowy windshield, I managed to plow about half-way up. The Subaru slowed, stopped. Four cylinders were just not enough. Wheels spun fruitlessly. I was stuck.

"Damn! damn! damn!" My expletives only served to fog up the windshield. *Such a hot shot you are, Cynthia. You goofed!* A burning flush swept up my body. Ted's negative predictions were coming true! The disapproving voice of Dad rang clearly in my ears: "Who do you think you are?" I hear that sometimes, when I fail.

What to do? Still hanging onto the illusion that I might get out of that pickle, I tried to back down. Since the drop-off side of the road was so scary, I over-compensated by hugging the other side— managing to slide slowly, silently, and elegantly into the ditch.

Tears came then, in the snowy silence, tears of frustration and humiliation. I was that child again, and Daddy was scolding me. I gave in to the old self pity. After indulging in it until the kid inside was satisfied, I wiped my eyes, blew my nose, grabbed my purse and struggled up out of the steeply tilted car onto the road.

Already somewhat weak from chemotherapy, mouth and esophagus sore, I slogged slowly up the hill; and, breathless, bewigged, red-nosed and red-eyed, knocked on Alton Christensen's door.

A hawk-beaked, bright-eyed giant of a man responded. Squawking raucously from his shoulder was a small, colorful, angry bird.

"Shush, Kechet," Alton admonished the bird. To me: "You must be Cynthia. Come on in." With a glance at the empty parking lot and my own disheveled appearance, he asked no questions, simply closed the door. Then he enfolded me in a bear hug that left me sobbing in relief.

"I ... I'm so sorry," I apologized, then blurted out my sad story.

"Was it your fault?" He asked me gently.

"Not exactly, but my husband didn't want me to come. I feel so stupid."

"Hmmm. Well, we'll work on that," he spoke softly. "But first, here's the telephone if you want to call Triple A to pull your car out."

I fumbled through my wallet and pulled out the AAA card. The print was so small I could hardly read it, even with my glasses on, especially with my hands still shaking. But finally arrangements were made to extricate the car, and I recovered enough to take stock of my surroundings.

Alton's house was a typical, cozy, small Santa Fe adobe with beamed ceilings and a cheerful fireplace. In what probably had been the dining area, under a skylight, stood a treatment table covered with Pendleton blankets. Two plump cats dozed comfortably on the sofa, oblivious to the bird's incessant chatter. Native American shamanic artifacts were on the walls and table by the window.

He motioned me to the couch and disappeared into the kitchen, returning with two glasses of raspberry juice.

"Here, drink this," he urged, handing me one.

"This tastes peculiar." I couldn't place the added flavor.

"Of course," he chuckled. "That's because I put trace minerals in it. Divine energy enters the body through trace minerals."

"Oh, OK." I sipped it gratefully, glad for incoming energy of any kind.

Kechet had obviously adopted Alton as her mate, for she hopped all over his arms and neck, pulled at his hair, nibbled at his ears and ate peanuts from his mouth—meanwhile throwing vituperative bird chatter at me, the intruder. Alton bore all this unwarranted attention with patience, continuing to supply peanuts to the unrelenting bird as we talked.

"Why don't you tell me a little about your life and why you are here?" he prompted. I gave him the capsule version, including daddy, the old sea captain, mom and husband number one.

Then he filled me in a little on his own background. He had been a medical doctor, a general practitioner, for a number of years; but began to feel he was not really curing people, only relieving the symptoms. Meanwhile he was being called to shamanism, and ignoring that call. The result was he went through agonies, even death experiences, before he finally got the message.

After a couple years as a healer in Brazil, where miracles occurred when he simply laid on hands and recited Catholic prayers, Alton returned to this country. Eventually he found himself in Santa Fe, successfully treating a number of people who had acute environmental illness. By word of mouth his practice there grew, until he finally decided to stay.

"You know," Alton suggested, "that in your case, as the tumor was on the right side of your body, your male side, it means that you have issues with the males in your life or the male energies within you."

"That sounds right," I confirmed. Though I still had unresolved issues with mother and sister, they did not feel hurtful. On the other hand, it had always been men who had controlled me. It's not that I hate men. On the contrary, growing up I liked them a lot, even preferred their company to women. It probably was to gain their approval. Still trying to get dad to love me. How foolish.

"Your father repressed your male energy," he continued, "and your passive mother taught you how to allow the male energy to be repressed, in order to survive."

Those words conjured up images of dad running things and mother floating along in the wake of his will. True. Never did she make decisions, and she seemed to like being treated that way because it gave her everything she wanted. No responsibility. Yes, Alton was right on that score.

"Furthermore," he continued, "people whose disease manifests on the side opposite their sex are healers."

This was beginning to sound like a one-two-three punch. I would have to give that notion some serious thought.

As we continued our conversation, Alton activated insights in rapid succession. A lot of hazy images from my early life suddenly came into clear focus. It was almost like he was pushing the right buttons to pop open hidden compartments, like a toy my two year old grandson plays with.

"I'll bet when that little girl was fondled by that old sea captain she just wanted to die of shame and humiliation," he cued me.

Oooh, yeah, I got the point. Had I really told some aspect of my psyche I wanted to die? Apparently I had, and the body was cooperating.

"Yes, but Alton, how do I change that?" I asked.

"In your meditation, go back to that time. Be the mother. Hold that child. Support her. Love her. Tell her she was not to blame. Offer to kick that old man in the groin, if necessary."

"Be the mother of myself, the child?"

"Yes. Support her, but let her do her own grieving. Be there, next to her, while she expresses her own emotions."

Yes, that child's voice had been screened for many, many years. I heard her when I wanted to play, have fun, watch sunsets, hike in the woods, body-surf in the ocean. But when it came to the old hurts, she didn't say a word. She must have been exceedingly well trained.

The roar of a truck's engine brought me out of my thoughts. Alton and I threw on our coats and boots to slide down the driveway, where the AAA truck was attempting to extricate the Subaru.

Oh no! We watched in horror as the truck slid into the ditch too. Now what?

An angry, frustrated driver climbed out of his cab, glaring at us and sputtering into his two way radio. "Yeah, I'm stuck. Come get me out."

"What about my car?"

"Sorry, lady, you'll have to wait until tomorrow."

Tomorrow? Spend the night here with this man I just met? Ted will be livid. "I told you so!" Hot flash. Burning cheeks. More guilt tightening the stomach. I decided to protest.

"Don't you have a four-wheel-drive tow truck?"

"Yes, but the boss won't send it out. Lady, this is a bad day. A hundred people are stuck."

We argued, but there was no changing anything, so Alton and I climbed back up the hill to the warm house and took off our wet coats and boots.

What was this lesson? I wondered. *Training in helplessness?*

Then a bright idea bubbled up to consciousness: Call another towing company and try to get Triple A to reimburse me. Alton was not making suggestions to rescue me. He was probably encouraging my "male" energy to act! So I looked up towing companies in the yellow pages and found a local one who would send out a four-wheel-drive truck in about an hour.

"Good," said Alton. "That will give us time for your treatment. Take off your socks and all your jewelry. You should have no metal on your body."

"Do you mind if I take off my wig?" I inquired, timidly. He looked puzzled. "It's acrylic." Someone had told me artificial fibers are bad for energy work, so I was wearing all cotton clothes.

"Oh, yes. Go ahead."

I went to the bathroom, left my wig on the sink and returned to the room bald. Alton didn't bat an eyelash.

Lying on the table, I looked up at the wooden beams and storm-gray skylight, while Alton covered me warmly and tenderly with a colorful Pendleton blanket.

He pressed some little silk pads into my hands, telling me to close my fists over them. Additional pads went under my neck and spine. Maybe they conducted energy?

Alton incarcerated a protesting Kechet, covered the cage, started a tape recording of soothing music and began rubbing my bare feet with fragrant oil. Oh my, it felt good! He pulled at each toe, cracking the joint. That felt good too. I closed my eyes and relaxed.

With one hand he touched my forehead, placing the other on the base of my skull. A few deep breaths and my shaman entered some other world. I began to tingle pleasantly from toes to head. As his hands moved to different parts of my body their warmth relaxed me further.

It was hard to let my mind go, because thoughts of the car kept intruding. In addition—a strange thing—I noticed part of me was observing all that was going on from a vantage point somewhere above and behind my right shoulder. Nevertheless, as time went on, the mind relaxed as well. I began to see beautiful colors behind closed eyelids.

Ooo! a sharp pain, as his gentle hands touched my right shoulder. *Wonder what that was about?*

Another sharp pain in the left ankle. *That's odd.*

"Let there be peace on earth and let it begin with me." *Where did that come from?* It just intruded into my mind. The melody and the words would not leave. Over and over they played. The part of me that was observing suggested it was a message to stop being anxious and radiate peace outward. So I just let the song flow on, and was finally filled with peacefulness.

A pressure of something cool on my solar plexus…*Gonnnnngggg!* The brass Tibetan bell's vibrations entered my body. As the sound faded away, I returned from that pleasant somewhere I had floated to.

"When you are ready, Cynthia," intoned Alton, "be awake and be present."

His footsteps faded, leaving the room. As my eyes opened, they were dazzled by sunshine pouring through the skylight. A purring cat was warming my feet on top of the blanket.

Alton returned from the bathroom laughing. "I see Moonshadow decided to share your journey."

I smiled sleepily. Moonshadow yawned, stretched and jumped down.

"Cynthia I must tell you, I sure was startled when I went into the bathroom. I thought it was Sunrise, the other cat, limply prostrate on the sink. It was your wig!" He walked over to the couch, still chuckling.

Amused at the thought, I dreamily sat up and climbed down off the table. All tension seemed to have left me.

"Alton," I remarked, putting on my jewelry and socks, "it feels as if there aren't any barriers left inside me— like I am hollow, and there is a warm, quiet river flowing through me."

He smiled knowingly. "That's lovely."

"Why did it hurt when you touched my shoulder and ankle?"

"That's where the memories are," he replied. "When I touched your right shoulder I could hear that child crying out in pain."

Again, truck noise interrupted our quiet talk. This time, as we emerged from the house and slid down the hill, the sun was shining brightly over a breathtaking panorama of snow-crowned, piñon-clad mountains and valleys.

At the site of my disaster, two highly skilled men were winching the car gently out of the ditch. With the greatest artistry, they turned it 180 degrees and drove it down to the bottom of the hill. Not a scratch on it! I paid them gratefully, then trekked back up for a few more minutes with Alton.

In those moments before I left, he gave me a tool for discovering more hidden parts of myself.

"Pretend you are in a familiar spot, like a restaurant. Observe every little detail, the sights, the smells, the sounds. Make it as real as possible.

Find yourself in conversation with someone and see who walks in and what those people say to you."

Then he hugged me, this great eagle/bear of a man, held me at arm's length, looked me straight in the eye, and said: "Above all, when you get home, don't let yourself be victimized." He repeated, shaking my shoulders gently for emphasis. "You must not allow yourself to be victimized."

Another quick hug, and I found myself joyfully negotiating the slippery driveway to my car, like a child in a snowy world of enchantment.

The drive home was no problem. By then the Interstate was cleared, but my thoughts were spinning around, repeating what Alton had told me. When I arrived, Ted was waiting anxiously. I told him the whole story of the ditch, and (Alton's voice echoing in my ears) did not allow myself to be a victim.

To my great surprise, I did not hear any I-told-you-so's. Amazing. And when I ate dinner, I realized my sore mouth and esophagus no longer hurt.

In the months, now years, since that day, Alton Christensen has been my teacher as well as my healer. With his permission, I am sharing just a few of his teachings that have been most helpful:

—"Consider your life here on earth to be a birth canal. It begins when you enter at birth, and ends with your death, your true birth. As you move along in that birth canal there will be polarities on either side of you. The trick is to not grab hold of either polarity, for it will hold up your progress. The baby will not emerge. So if on one side you have joy and the other sorrow, do not hold onto either of them. You must balance the polarities, thus neutralizing them, so you can continue to move along."

—"Forgiveness is not necessarily the proper reaction to a hurt of the inner child. If you were to come home and the baby sitter has beat up your child, outrage would be a more appropriate emotion. Forgiveness, in the sense of understanding the message inherent in the hurt, releasing it later, and recognizing only oneness on a spiritual plane, is a transformative process."

—"When you have physical or emotional pain, go into that pain. Experience it as much as possible, then be very still and let it talk to you, to give you its message."

—"You must not ignore limiting beliefs, you must work through them, exposing them for what they are, illusion. All mental programming is illusion too, but it serves an educational purpose."

—"We begin in unity with Divinity, but lose our sense of identity with it as we come to the earth plane. As we climb higher in our path, we come closer to unity again; so the Divine figures more prominently in our lives. Little miracles, peeks behind the curtains, synchronicities, happen more frequently."

—"Since we cannot see ourselves as divine in our conscious mind, we put those images into our subconscious. From there we project them out as images separated from ourselves. Everything we see as separate from ourselves is really a projection of ourselves from our unconscious mind."

—"Externalizing is giving someone else your power."

—"Crisis may be necessary to achieve transformation. Crisis cuts us loose from being so terribly grounded in this reality that we do not perceive our true identity."

—"As we grow, we come back to the same place again and again. Yet because we always make progress it is not a circle, but a spiral. This process does not stop with our death, but continues over and over, spiraling upwards towards enlightenment, or oneness with our Divinity, through many lifetimes and many levels of understanding."

—"The only sin is failure to grow."

—"The body has the power to heal itself, but people have to clear out the psychological issues that cause the illness before healing can take place."

—"Disease occurs because the body, being the densest layer of our being, is where issues are placed on a cellular level to be worked out. You don't ask the school superintendent to change a light bulb. You ask the janitor. The body tries to resolve issues we bury there, and the result is disease. That is why so much illness is metaphoric in nature. Sexual abuse results in disease of the sexual parts, buried anger results in ulcers (I can't stomach this!), or colitis results from trying to compete for attention by perfection (I don't have any intestinal fortitude)."

—"Healing is a process. It does not usually occur in a blinding flash because we have stuffed so much into our body on that cellular level. As we uncover one thing, we can move on to others."

—"Cancer of the left breast is often associated with lack of nurturing and bonding with the mother. Cancer of the right breast is often unresolved issues with the animus."

—"The greatest suffering is the greatest opportunity, because from pain comes transformation."

—"The positive side of incest, since all things have polarity, is that it brings forth the divine child."

—"We must transform suffering and sickness. Between polarities lies the energy to lift one's self out of the victim position and into the position of power. Polarities create energy because of the interaction between them. The gap, the space between, the void, the womb, is where the shaman works."

It is inherent in the character of teachings that we understand them more fully as we progress in awareness. Take, for instance, the concept of sharing. To a toddler, sharing may mean one cookie for me, one for her. An older child may incorporate in his concept of sharing breaking the cookie in half and giving half to another child, accepting less to benefit another. For an adolescent, sharing may expand to include the concept of spending time with other people to create a project or help with homework.

As we become adults, we begin to understand that sharing also means giving from the heart. We come to know that sharing does not mean dividing, but expanding. Like love, for instance. You can love your first child one hundred percent. You can love each subsequent child one hundred percent as well. It just expands.

An interesting corollary would be that the more you love, the more capacity for love you develop. And, in polarity, the more you hate, the more capacity you have for hating.

The basic structure of a concept takes on more complexity with each new level of growth and understanding. Every time I met with my shaman I added a new layer of awareness.

The curious part is that each addition of new awareness resulted in the subtraction of an old layer of garbage. Metaphysical mathematics. I wish they taught that kind of math in schools.

Occasionally, Alton's extra sensory perception startled me. Like the time he glanced up as I was walking normally into the house and said, "You have something wrong with your left hip. There is pain there—I can see it in your aura."

He was right, naturally. I had been having a lot of pain in that area for weeks. When I walked out two hours later, the pain was gone.

Each laying on of hands was a little different. Alton says he just asks Divine Mother what to do and she tells him. There were times it seemed I floated above my body. Sometimes energy waves sent shivers through my whole physical being. Other times I saw colors and geometric shapes—or entered the emptiness of the void, the place of nothingness, pregnant with potential.

Some strange, mysterious things also happened in the "real" world, such as the time he paid special attention to my "third eye" in the middle of my forehead. Driving home, a thunderstorm deluged the car. When it cleared, the windshield had a huge crack directly in front of my forehead. Nothing had hit it.

But perhaps the most significant moment, a turning point in my healing, was when he reprogrammed me.

"Cynthia, do you think you really can be completely healed?" he asked one day.

Taken aback, I stammered "I, I think I can."

"Let's see if you really mean it. Raise your arm and resist my pressure after you say, 'I think I can be completely healed.'"

I resisted his hand pushing down my arm, as hard as I could.

"Now say, 'I do *not* think I can be completely healed.'"

This time my resistance was just a little stronger, but not enough to be significant.

"You are ambivalent about it," he declared. "Let's reprogram you." He taught me a ritual that consisted of tapping my middle finger against a certain spot in my other hand and repeating "I believe I can be completely healed" over and over, aloud and to myself. It sounds strange, almost like "The Little Engine Who Could," but there is an energy path rationale behind it.

Betty tells me she remembers that is when the great fear left me.

I can truthfully tell you that afterwards it was easier to be positive, and I really believed—strange as it may seem—that despite all the medical nay-saying, despite the gloom and doom of tests and pathology reports, I was going to get well. Completely.

And I did.

The call to shamanism is little understood, especially in our Western culture; and it is often misinterpreted by the person who is called.

It flies in the face of all our perceptions—especially confronting the "myth" of materialism. The myth is that our material world is defined by the boundaries of our five senses.

In actuality, we can perceive only a tiny share of the data "out there." If one is open to the idea that reality exists beyond our capacity to be aware of it, then the concepts of shamanism are less exotic.

In more "primitive" cultures, a person being called to shamanism may easily understand what is happening to him or her; but the average American would begin to doubt his own sanity.

Such a person, unaware of his calling, was Alton Christensen. His path to shamanism followed a tortuous route through crisis, to the point of apparent physical death. There were other deaths as well: relationships, ego, preconceptions; and finally surrender to a greater will. It was this surrender that unlocked the gates restraining him from moving forward in his preordained vocation.

Death and rebirth are the classic way of the shaman. Death and rebirth create transformation. The healer who has been wounded is better able to help others who suffer from their own wounds. This is an ancient calling, dating from the beginnings of humanity.

Alton always knew that he was going to be a healer, but he assumed he would be a doctor, in the way our culture defined a healer. So he went to medical school, graduating *cum laude* from the University of Colorado School of Medicine in 1972. He interned at Butterworth Hospital in Grand Rapids, Michigan, and went on to practice family medicine in Oregon, from 1973 to 1980.

By the time I interviewed Alton for this book, he had moved from his little home in Tesuque to a modern town house in Santa Fe. No more treacherous driveway!

Many previously stored belongings now graced his tables, windows and walls. As I sat in a commodious living room chair drinking apple juice, Alton stretched out on a couch facing me. We were surrounded by huge amethyst and quartz crystals, earth spirit sculpture, unique shamanic artifacts, stained glass, paintings and various other art objects. It was a rich and sacred space.

Moonshadow and Sunrise slept in total oblivion near French doors opening to a Santa Fe style patio. Through the glass I could see sheltering autumn foliage splash sunshine onto the earthen tile floor and wooden benches.

Kechet, Alton informed me, had fallen in love with another bird and gone to live with him. Presumably she was happy at last with someone of her own species. In her absence the room was quiet and peaceful.

We talked comfortably about this and that, just a couple of friends sharing news. Gradually, the conversation drifted into the reasons why Alton had left his successful medical practice.

"I was very busy in the practice of medicine at the time," he mused, "and very disappointed in it. Very unhappy with where I found myself."

"Why was that?" It runs contrary to our image of doctors to think of them as unhappy in their profession.

"Because I was realizing that there were very few modalities within the framework of allopathic medicine that were healing or transformative. Most treatments were suppressive.

"You know, we see advertisements on TV where someone says 'I have a terrible headache,' and they take an aspirin. Then they smile and say, 'I don't have a headache any more!' The fact is, they still have their headache—they have just blocked the perception of the headache.

"We know from Framingham studies and many other medical studies that you can take people with chronic diseases such as hypertension and diabetes, whose symptoms are kept under control for decades, and when the organs are examined *post mortem,* tissue damage has proceeded as if there had been no treatment whatsoever.

"This is true of much of medicine. A large portion of general practice is prescriptions, prescribing medicines for whatever ailments the person has. There is very little that is effective in a transforming way, a curative way, for the individual.

"I was becoming aware of other studies, too, at that time. I had attended a conference in which a fellow from London was talking about the research that had been done with mongoloids.

"Mongoloids are mentally retarded, right? They score very, very low on IQ testing. Somebody realized that the IQ testing only regards the left hemisphere of the brain; it doesn't regard the right. So he took a group of mongoloid third graders—eight year olds—and allowed them certain experiences imprinting the right hemisphere in alternative relation to the left. After a few months he put them in normal third grade classes. By the end of the nine month school year, the mongoloids excelled. They were superior in their performance to the normal controls in third grade—and fourth grade too!"

"In all the class work?" That sounded unbelievable.

"All the work, not just right-brained work," he confirmed.

"In another instance, one of my woman patients had gone to visit relatives in California and suffered a massive stroke there. She entered a hospital specializing in neurology and underwent months and months of intensive physical therapy. When she finally came back to Oregon, one arm was flaccidly paralyzed. It was like a wet old rag. She walked with a cane, supported on the other side by her husband, because one leg was substantially involved as well.

"I decided to take the mongoloid technique and modify it for her. I asked her to read something interesting before she went to bed—something that would capture her attention, not too familiar so that it would be boring, nor too complicated so that it would be frustrating. She was to read for 45 minutes of the last hour before bedtime. For the last 15 minutes, the lights were to be off and she was to be tucked into bed, listening to non-verbal music.

"The London research showed that every time you engage the left hemisphere of the brain, and then immediately afterwards do something to affect the right hemisphere, the two hemispheres begin to engage. They begin to connect in a very meaningful way. It's like they mirror each other, and see where the other needs some support or some substitution in function. They take over for each other.

"This, in effect, is what I asked her to do. To facilitate the process I had her take a small dose of DNA/RNA for a few days one week, a few days the next week, and that was the end of it.

"After two or three months of this bedtime regimen, she returned to full function. The arm became totally normal, and the leg also.

"It was a bit of fresh air. But it was also outside of what was approved by the AMA, or standard medical practice.

"Those were a couple of inspiring moments in what was for me a rather depressing practice, because of the suppressive nature of medicine. I was very, very disappointed, because my goal had been to serve in a much more meaningful way."

The cases he talked about seemed almost like miracles. More was at work, obviously, than pills and drugs. "Was this the beginning of your move into shamanism?" I asked.

"It's hard to pinpoint the beginning," he responded, "but events just sort of kept occurring that started giving me a clue. Two years after I began practicing medicine, I took my family to Mexico, where I became very ill with diarrhea. Besides that, I had severe breathing difficulties, so it clearly wasn't the usual traveler's diarrhea—but what it was, nobody knew.

"A week after I returned home I began to experience two very serious problems. One was a total inability to sleep, and the other was bright red rectal bleeding. Gushing, serious bleeding, accompanied by an ache in the cecum. Doctors told me it was not possible, because a lesion producing bright red bleeding would have to be further down in the intestinal tract.

"I went to many doctors to try to identify the bleeding, but they were blocked by this allopathic framework of what they had been taught in medical school. Nobody could figure out what was wrong. In addition to allopathic medicine not serving the needs of my patients, it was clearly not serving me.

"At the end of 1979 I was given only a few months to live. Nobody could figure out why I had been bleeding since mid-1975, and unable to sleep in the same period of time. In early January of 1980 I went to the sleep disorders clinic in Palo Alto, and they were asking me why I had survived for so long. I had no idea why I was still alive.

"Later that month I underwent exploratory surgery. They found I had a genetic disease, Osler-Weber-Rendu syndrome, which weakens the walls of veins in the gut and elsewhere, producing bleeding.

"They said that nothing could be done. Here again is a place where allopathic medicine isn't serving. The framework is 'Here is a genetic disease, therefore it's the way it is, and one can't do anything about it.'

"The next part is a little hard for most people to believe, Cynthia, so you may not even want to put it in writing."

My curiosity gave him full attention. I grabbed my pen.

"Two months after the surgery I took my family to Hawaii. The decision to go was made quickly, so I had no time to get traveler's checks. I sent my nurse June down to the bank with a check to get cash, so I had a large amount of cash. In the evening after we arrived, I went down to the beach to walk and relax.

"At that time I was into materialism as compensation for the low self esteem that I carried from my childhood wounds. So I had a four-teen-karat gold Rolex watch. On a solid gold chain that had been insured by Lloyds of London I carried a ring with a diamond valued at about $100,000. I had stuffed about $2500 cash in each sock, and had several hundred dollars in my billfold.

"In addition, at the other end of the scale, I had a wedding ring that cost probably twenty dollars, because I was married upon graduating from medical school and at that time twenty dollars was a lot. Oh yes, I also had a medical school class ring that was probably worth sixty-five bucks.

"That's what I had on me when I decided to go for that walk along Waikiki Beach, about quarter to seven in the evening.

"At midnight, two Navy officers who were patrolling the harbor noticed my body in the water. They pulled me out and called an ambu-lance. I was informally pronounced dead on the beach, taken to Queens Hospital, officially pronounced dead in the emergency room and taken to the morgue.

"Around six or seven in the morning, a resident on his way to work took a short cut through the morgue. As he was passing by my body, which was on a cart, an inner male voice (he later reported) said to him, 'Put your stethoscope on that body.' He was an atheist, but he heard that voice three times, and the third time he heard it, he said it was a com-mandment he had to obey.

"So he did. After a while he thought he heard a heartbeat, so they rushed me up to intensive care. They found drug metabolites in my urine, but I never took drugs.

"It had been a robbery. Oddly, although the cash in my socks was gone, my wedding ring and the Rolex watch too, they did not take my class ring, the cash in my billfold or the chain with the ring around my neck. Of an approximate total value of $110,000, ten percent was taken. Isn't it peculiar?"

The ten percent rang a bell immediately. "It was a tithe!" I declared.

"Yes. Years later I was able to remember being held on the edge of a large boat that night and having convulsive seizures, held down by two guys while a third guy was stuffing something down my throat. I actually was able to relive the drowning, the feeling of taking water into the lungs, to a total surrender."

"What a horrible experience!" My own breathing labored in sympathy. I've had a fear of drowning ever since David Smith held me under water until I nearly ran out of air, when we were children. He says he was only trying to kiss me. Sure, he was. (But he's still my friend.)

"There was symbolism in my experience too," Alton continued, reaching down to pet Moonshadow, who had arisen for the sole purpose of receiving strokes. "I looked at the nature of what was stolen. The five grand was gone—there was just enough money left for us to get out of Hawaii.

"The wedding ring was gone. I was not to have any more marriage and family. I knew that in some way that was not clear at the time. And the watch was gone. I knew I had no more time, but did not know what that meant either.

"So, although I had a certain awareness since I was very little, I came out of Hawaii sort of knowing things in a new way."

I sipped my apple juice thoughtfully. "Did you understand then you were being called to shamanism?"

"No, not really. More had to happen first." Moonshadow jumped off the couch and came over to me, purring and rubbing up against my leg. Alton smiled and resumed his narrative while I scratched her ears.

"When I came back from Hawaii there was a letter in my mailbox from a lady I had treated for some sort of arthritis. I had only seen her a couple times, and yet here was this very personal letter from her. She spoke about hovering over the operating table in January when I was undergoing exploratory surgery, and she related things I alone knew from conversations with the doctor, and which I had told nobody.

"I myself was an agnostic in those days, Cynthia, but I thought, *There's something here*, and called her up. She came over and told me of her connection with a healing center run by two Benedictine nuns. She worked there a couple times a week, laying on hands. The center's name was Shalom, and I began going there to receive healing—but they always had me work as a healer, even though I did not know what I was doing.

"I had closed my practice the first day of January, 1980, because of my illness. The end of March, after returning from Mexico, I moved out of my home, to an apartment in Portland. I began working on securities investments to make money.

"In that apartment, one afternoon, I had a terrifying experience."

"What happened?"

"I was lying down on the living room couch resting, when in through the ceiling (I was on the seventh floor of a fourteen story apartment building) flew a bird that was an eagle. I knew she was a female, although I don't know how I knew it.

"She flew down as if she were picking up a prey and thrust her talons into my chest wall. Blood spurted from the holes, and the pain felt like it was occurring physically. It was like someone had taken a hammer and driven thick nails into my chest!

"It was extraordinary pain, and horror—because from my early childhood history of being abused I had a lot of body insecurity issues, body integrity issues.

"She thrust her talons into my chest and then she lifted me off, which was also incredibly painful, and we went through the ceiling as though the ceiling were a vapor."

"This was in what dimension?" I inquired incredulously.

"I couldn't really tell you. Anyway we flew off as if the ceiling were a cloud, not a tangible, limiting object. We flew off to a cliffside. There with her beak she began ripping the flesh from my bones. All of this was as physically painful as if it were happening in this reality, and psychologically—again, because of the earlier history—very traumatic."

"I'll bet!"

"I was caught up in the horror of this experience. I was engulfed in it. When she had stripped all the flesh from my bones she went right through my calvarium, the dome of my skull, and began pulling out my brains.

"At that moment it sort of flipped. I realized I was alive, and the whole horror fell into comic relief. That ended the experience. As you can imagine, I had no framework for this kind of happening."

"I'll bet you didn't!" If my comments were banal, it was because all verbal ability had been squelched by vividly imagining the scene.

"My only framework was traditional medicine, and in that framework I concluded I had a psychotic break."

"That would be a reasonable assumption to make."

Alton laughed. "I was not ever going to tell that story to anybody, for any reason. It was not until much later that I learned it is a classic shamanic dismemberment motif and part of the process.

"But after this experience, the Christ became visually available to me. I would not see him physically as tangibly as I see you, or I presume you see me, but like an apparition. I would converse with him similarly to what we are doing here.

"Sometimes we would walk by a river in a desert and he would teach. The teachings had to do with the purpose or constructive function of illness—whether it be illness of the physical body or of the mind, emotions, or spirit.

"Sometimes he would take me with him. When he was about to take me I always knew, because my body would become extremely fatigued. I would stop whatever I was doing and lie down. My spirit would leave and join him. We would go places, look at organ systems, relationship conflicts, all sorts of levels of problems, OK?"

"OK." I was still reduced to monosyllables.

"And the symbolic message behind the illness. He taught that the illness has within it a way through the illness, in the transformation of the particular illness, OK?"

"OK."

"In all of this I questioned. It was all very curious in some ways---"

"Nice to have your own special teacher," I interjected, not intending to sound sarcastic.

"---and yet, deep within myself was, *This is all just insanity. This is some hallucinatory function of the mind.*"

"Well, this is how it would be perceived by most people." I stirred uncomfortably, wondering how many people might be in mental institutions who were really seers into some other worlds.

Alton got up from the couch, took my glass and went into the kitchen to refill it with apple juice. I took a few deep breaths, trying to integrate these amazing stories with my view of reality. By this time, I knew there are other existences beyond our three-dimensional world, but the narrative issuing so easily from Alton's lips flowed like a screen play. Still and all, knowing the man, I believed him.

I drank from the glass he brought back. Alton was in high gear. The story continued to unfold effortlessly. "One day the Christ said to me, 'You're to go to Brazil to help a young man.'

"I was expecting a vision of what this guy looked like, and when I didn't get one, I asked the Christ to tell me what he looked like. There was no response. I said, 'What is his name?' and even went so far as to say 'Do you realize that Brazil is a large country? I could be missing this guy by a couple blocks in a big city and hunt there for a few centuries and not find him.' This was the state of my own funniness, you see. At which point the Christ completely disappeared from view. He would not appear again.

"So now I did not know what to do. In a conversation with my investment partner, I said, 'I've been thinking about taking a little vacation.' He said, 'Have you ever been to Brazil?' And I thought to myself, *This is interesting.*

"Within five minutes he made a telephone call and introduced me to a young man named Claudio in Sao Paulo, who spoke English. So now I knew who to see and where to go. I just called a travel agent and said 'Book me on a plane to Sao Paulo September 13.'

"I arrived at the hotel room in Brazil expecting the Christ to meet me there, as if he had booked an earlier plane, if you will! I was disappointed, frustrated, and once again the old story played to me— *This is just madness, this is insanity. I have lost it and I don't even know it. This is crazy!*

"I tried to calm myself, took a shower and went downstairs. It was like automatic walking. I stopped at the gift shop just as it was closing and bought a little Portuguese/English dictionary, then walked out into the streets. I walked a few blocks, then saw the steeple of a church. I was connecting with Shalom, it was a Catholic Center, and with all this calling into Shamanism, it occurred to me that might be where I was going to meet the young man I came to Brazil to help.

"When I approached the big doors, I saw they were locked with heavy chains. 'Oh, Christ!' I swore, and turned my head to see in the shadows a young man sitting on a rock in the position of that thinking man that the sculptor--- What's the name of it?"

"Rodin. *The Thinker.*"

"Yes, that was it. When I saw him the Christ reappeared and said, 'That's the man you came to help.' "

"Cool."

"And so it instilled in me a lot of things, not only trust, but the beginning of an understanding that this was something far more than a psychotic break, right?"

"Sure, because you were given reinforcement. It worked. One thing led to another, and it worked."

"Does that give you a kind of an answer to your question?"

I giggled. "Yes indeed. If all that happened to me, it would probably land me in the loony bin!"

After thinking about it a moment, I changed my mind. "Actually, if that happened to me now I would work at seeing the guidance being given. If it happened a few years ago I would have thought I was going crazy."

"Yes," he agreed.

"So is it appropriate to assume that was the beginning point of your career as a shaman? Were you not called upon to do something specific working with people in Brazil?"

"Yes, I was. The young man's name was Jair. He came from an impoverished rural background, an alcoholic, abusive father, and needing work, had come to the big city to find it. He had been there three days without food, no place to sleep. Tired, hungry and desperate, he had come to the church to ask for guidance. The interfacing of these two stories, you see, is awesome."

I agreed.

Alton continued his story. "We went to his home town in southern Brazil. There we stayed with his family. The next morning, his mother, Lazara, is frying eggs at the stove and I'm sitting at a little kitchen table and she rubs the right side of her rear end. I ask her what is the matter and she says 'Arthritis.' So I kneel down on the floor while she fries her eggs and I plaster my hands on her rump and say my Catholic prayers! I didn't know what the hell was going on.

"Jair and I ate our eggs and went on a long journey by foot. We did not get home until about 6:30 that night. Soon after starting out, I took a step with my right leg and almost fell to the sidewalk. The pain in my hip was extraordinary. I didn't associate it with the fact I had just worked on Lazara. It was her pain, and I had taken it on, but I didn't understand that then.

"I was very sick at the time. I had not slept for nearly five years, I was still bleeding internally and rectally, and I was in the early stages of getting bilateral pneumonia. Now I have the addition of this right hip pain and I say to the Christ, 'You know, I'm really carrying enough!' He only looks at me with a lot of love.

"At the end of this long day, I am limping back home with Jair. Lazara, very intuitive, knows we are coming over the horizon. She's out there in the middle of the street, her arms are up to the sky and she is smiling with joy. Her arthritis is gone.

"The moment I see her I know it's her hip pain in me, and I struggle for the next three days trying to get it out. I can't even tell you how it was ultimately discharged, but after about seventy-two hours it just went 'tooq' and it was gone.

"Lazara's healing brought lots of people, lines and lines of people wanting to be cured. One woman came to me with her ten year old daughter, who had an obvious goiter. The underactive thyroid was never treated, so she became mentally retarded. They put her in a regular school so she would learn some social skills, but that situation severely eroded her self esteem. She was the last of a long line of people needing healing.

"I was running a high fever with the pneumonia; I was totally exhausted. But I put my hands on her and said ten minutes of Catholic prayers. That was it. There wasn't anything more I could give to anybody.

"That night Jair and I rode the bus back to Sao Paulo. The following day I took a plane to the United States. It wasn't until five years later that I returned back to Brazil, where I was greeted by the same girl, now fifteen years old. I couldn't believe her story. She was a straight-A student, and the most artistically gifted child in the school. I had to get other people to corroborate what she told me, for even though I had witnessed many healings, I had never seen anything so dramatic. From powerlessness comes empowerment. She was mentally retarded; this was the flip-flop of that."

"That's quite a story."

The sun was sliding lower, sending long shadows into the room where we were conversing. I didn't want to interrupt Alton, because his narrative seemed to flow meaningfully from one event to the next. Any questions I might ask would only divert and fracture it.

"She was not an isolated case. She was one of hundreds. Hundreds of people were cured, and how I did that I did not know. In fact, I would say to myself repeatedly, 'This is some sort of placebo function. They are really hysterics, they are really hypochondriacs, there's nothing really wrong with them.' I didn't know what was going on."

"You just laid your hands on people and said Catholic prayers and somehow they got better."

"And somehow they got better," he agreed. "My plan was to set up a healing center in Brazil, but after my return to the United States, Brazil became ever more distant.

"I think what I was learning from all this—my own illness and my healing of others—in an experiential way, was what the earlier teachings from the Christ were about. That is, the treasure that's in an illness."

I could sense another story beginning.

"I remember one fellow, a couple of years ago, who came to me with a diagnosis of multiple sclerosis from a California neurologist. For four years his arm had been held up against his chest, frozen in place. His father, a test pilot, had blown up in a plane when he was nine years old.

"He was Jewish. In the Jewish faith there is a lot of devaluation of the feminine. Sometimes women get hostile when they have to deal with so much devaluation. So they sometimes take out reprisal in a vengeful way. What his mother did when his father died was conceptually castrate him. She made him docile, helpless, dependent, certainly not assertive. None of his masculine forces were being nourished or defined for him. He grew up with the most odious hate for women.

"He and his wife arrived. I lived in Tesuque up on this hill behind the fire station, and the driveway up the hill was quite treacherous."

"Oh! I know!"

"In the winter, people sometimes—"

"Sometimes go in the ditch!"

"Uh huh," he smiled. I laughed out loud.

"On this particular occasion it was raining and dark in the very late afternoon. She drove down the hill while I was working with him. It was very, very clear to me in the dialogue part of the shamanic work that this guy was emotionally castrated. This is a very loaded issue to talk about with a man. He was a professor at a university near San Clemente. He was heading back there in a day or two, and would be gone for nine months.

"I was seeing him one time only, and I was rather reluctant to bring out a heavily charged issue like that, so I just laid aside the issue and worked on him energetically. Of course, when he got up, everything was the same, right? I think he's not going to be too disappointed with this because he's from an allopathic framework, right? Well, not so.

"We wait and wait, and finally the lady arrives and knocks on the door. She just cowers in the doorway, wringing her hands, and looking like a dog laying on its back about to be chewed apart by a bigger dog.

" 'I'm so *sorry*, Dr. Christensen, I'm just *so sorry*.' When I asked her what happened, she explained that the car had gone in the ditch because on her way up—you know it's a little slippery, but there's this fantastic mountain vista, right? And she's looking over there and the car gets stuck on the right side.

"She calls AAA from the house, and they can't get here for an hour, or hour and a half."

"This is sounding awfully familiar!"

"So I know I'm going to have to deal with his psychological story. The three of us sat down and very gently I began looking at his history. Neurologically, although it was classical multiple sclerosis according to allopathic medicine, it was localized to the left side.

"What I was hearing from my guidance was there was a terrific amount of rage, anger, resentment against women. He reveals this because when she is at the door begging in apology, he gets up with his cane and [Alton is acting this out.] his face tenses up, and his voice was like this [strained, muffled, angry]. Then he relaxes and says 'Oh well, there must be a reason for it.' [Now Alton becomes docile and resigned.] He shoves it all back in.

"He's learned the teaching from a fellow named Gurdjieff who says there is always a positive reason for what happens. So if someone side-swipes him running a stop sign, he won't get angry, because it happened for a good reason."

I groaned. I've heard that, and I've said that. "This is a subtle trap we can fall into easily."

"I knew very little about him, but I knew where his rage was coming from. It had to do with his feminine side, his left side, because the paralysis was there. So we went through the whole castration issue, and how that happened. His wife could affirm, and she did many times in the next hour and a half, how that happened.

"When they finally had their car out of the ditch, he stood up from the couch and his arm dropped to the side, like a rag. It had been stiff up against his chest. He looked at it, extended his fingers and his palm, looked at me and said, 'You know, I haven't been able to do this in four years!'

"That was the symbolic message of his particular disease, which scientifically was labeled multiple sclerosis. In allopathic medicine, there is no cure for it. It's usually progressive and degenerative. So here is a place where the 'incurable' can be moved into a framework that allows a healing, allows a transformation."

This is an extraordinarily hopeful point of view. I have a friend with multiple sclerosis who believes everything the doctors tell her. I hope she reads this, and explores a little on her own.

"Alton, do you believe that there is a symbolic message in every disease?"

He spoke slowly and deliberately. "There is a symbolic message in every disease."

"I have seen the X-rays, for instance, of the fellow with scoliosis that you healed. What was the symbolic message?"

"Scoliosis is another thing that has a kind of family tree. It's an inherited disorder. People with scoliosis incarnate into a family that cannot, or will not, emotionally or psychologically support them. So what the child does is abdicate his own being-ness, and then takes on whatever the parents want him to be. He 'screws' or 'corkscrews' himself into what the parents want the child to be. And so the 'unscrewing' of the scoliotic spine has to do with identifying this as a problem, and identifying the examples in his own history where he sold himself off to what somebody else wanted him to be.

"Then one gives him techniques and tools for actually setting the mental body in a framework that is not going to buy into the same story. The transformation of scoliosis also includes accessing the DNA molecule and shifting its molecular structure. As in the case of the fellow with multiple sclerosis, this was a very clear mental body problem. Yet it's a far more encompassing thing because it involves a continuum of being-ness. It's spirit, mind, emotions and physical body. I'm not suggesting that all multiple sclerosis issues are only mental body. This is just one story, and each person has his or her own unique story."

I saw this as an opportunity to couple Alton's fascinating history to my journey. Scratching the tip of my nose with my pen (why do noses itch when you are thinking hard?) I said, "That's what I was going to ask you about breast cancer. I was going to ask you if you saw a symbolic message in breast cancer."

He shook his head, indicating it wasn't as simple as all that.

"Everyone is very, very unique." After a moment's thought he continued, "I believe this is another part of the problem—that we come with our preconceived understandings. For instance, a person can have a bacterial problem like pneumonia. You can blanket people with penicillin to take care of most of them, so we have a general statement that we apply to the individual case.

"But in spiritual unfolding, the individual is absolutely unique. So it behooves us to get the person's story, and really get a sense of its application to that particular being.

"There are some general, entry level statements that serve to work in the beginning, to sort of open the doors. You have to look at the childhood relationships, for example.

"I remember working with a very gifted healer who had aggressive, invasive breast cancer. She was born into a very wealthy and talented family. Her mother, who had a beautiful voice, was sent all over the world to study with the great masters; but as she matured she became a schizophrenic and was unable to give her daughter the nurturing the daughter needed.

"Being into the holistic stuff, the woman refused surgical intervention. She went instead to the Gersham Clinic and got on this healthy diet program. A few years later she saw a shaman from San Francisco whom I knew, and that shaman asked me to help.

"I went to see her. The cancer was in her left breast. In her case, the left breast was her feminine breast, so I knew the issue was with her mother. Schizophrenic people don't have a real ability to relate to someone else in an emotional or feeling tone way, so I knew she had not gotten the necessary bonding with the mother. She internalized this deep resentment.

"In internalizing the deep resentment, she carried in the cells the negative side of the disease's function. Everything has a negative and a positive side. We don't want to get too lopsided on one side or the other, or else we usually fall off a cliff somewhere.

"She was caught up in the negative side, the unforgiveness side, of her mother's inability to nurture. It's like victims who like being victims. They would not admit to being victims, but they stay in the victim mode for years and years and years and years. They are caught up in it because society is very cruel and punishing to the other side of the victim, which is the victimizer."

I nodded, my face flushing, very aware of how easy it is to be a victim and how hard to balance it by standing up for oneself. In the victim's mind, standing up for your rights often equates to being a victimizer—that is, hurting someone's feelings. And hurting someone's feelings is something from which we suffer extreme guilt.

"Although she was a gifted healer herself," Alton continued, acknowledging my awareness with his eyes, "she did not honor the constructive side of the wound. She didn't understand her healing gift being the rose that grows out of the compost pile.

"In that session I was able to get her very deeply into the pain of the lack of nurturing by her mother and the deep unexpressed resentment that she carried. She felt the hurt she had never felt before.

"It was interesting, because a week or two before I had that session with her she had a regular mammogram. With all her diet and meditations and searching within herself, growing and healing, the tumor, though it had been diagnosed as invasive, always stayed the same size. A week following this session with me she had another mammogram, and the tumor had shrunk twenty-five percent. We had accessed a part of that tumor.

"So I think as a general statement one can look at a symbolic function of an organ system. Kidneys represent how we psychologically mediate our way through life.

"Let's say you were born and raised in a Catholic family. Mom was Catholic and Dad was probably Baptist but signed up for the Catholic church as sort of an obligation, so your primary teachings of Catholicism are from your mother. And now, as part of your spiritual unfolding you are supposed to get into Buddhism, or Mormonism, or Lutheranism—it doesn't matter what. Insofar as you might have difficulty releasing the Catholic teaching, you would begin to compromise the function of the left (feminine side) kidney.

"So you can begin to understand some general sense of symbolism. Then we can get into the person's own individual history, which will shed light on what the uniqueness is."

He stopped, turning his head to face the French doors to the patio, waiting for my next question. It wasn't exactly a question, more of an observation.

"I assume this is the purpose of the dialogue you establish with your clients; the first part of the two-part healing session. The first part is a dialogue and the second part is a laying on of hands."

"There are several reasons for the dialogue. One is that, even though the way in which I experience a person's energy field gives me the information I need about that individual, I'm interested in how the person's mortal life is discordant with his or her energy.

"For instance, if the person understands that Catholicism is the 'right' religion, but if the energy field says that Buddhism is right for the client, then I'll talk to them a lot about their religion, to see if there is a place where they might align themselves, bring themselves into harmony with all levels of their being-ness.

"Another reason for the dialogue is if a person is intentionally lying about something, the energy field jolts in a peculiar way that informs me he's not telling me the truth, and he knows he's not telling me the truth. It reacts in a different way if he thinks he's telling me the truth, but he's not. It doesn't move at all if he is telling the truth, and he knows he's telling the truth."

A kind of extra sensory lie detector test, I thought. *Very useful.* "So the dialogue gives you the opportunity to match what you perceive in the energy field to what the person is experiencing in real life," I reiterated.

"Yes. It's not to find out where people are lying, you see---"

He picked up my thought! Was it in my aura?

"---but it's to identify where people understand something that really is a misunderstanding."

I was humbled. "They are not in harmony with themselves," I ventured, by way of smoothing things over.

"They are not in harmony with themselves," Alton calmed the waters, proceeding without interruption.

"If there is framing to be done—like the mental body is sitting in a position that's counter-productive to the physical body, then the mind has to be reframed so that it's not going to continue the program.

"The difficult reality is that the body speaks a different language than the mind. It's almost as if the mind speaks English and the body understands Chinese. So the mind can tell the body in English all it wants to tell the body, but the body absolutely cannot respond. The cellular program has to be shifted. I told you that little programming thing to do."

"Little? It changed my life!"

Alton sailed on, unheedful of my little ripple. "But on the other hand, if the mind continues a way of belief that is destructive to physical well-being, it does very little good to shape-shift the body into a new state of being and have a mind, then, that is still discordant. Then the being-ness is still out of balance."

I am thinking hard, trying to keep up with him. I had given up on taking notes a while back, just relying on the tape recorder. My mind couldn't keep up while my hand was working. It's always like this with Alton. The front part of my forehead gets tired when I talk with him, from thinking, like a muscle that has had a good workout.

"You can look upon a person as having a spirit body, a mental body, an emotional body, and a physical body. Four levels, right? If a person goes off and cleans up three of the four vehicles, leaving one bereft— such as the emotional body full of all sorts of unexpressed hurt, suffering and rage—then the emotional body will have to intensify its darkness to keep the life in total balance.

"Because physical life always achieves balance. The dark will always come in to balance the light. If you clean up three of the four vehicles, you will create an imbalance in the total life that will be balanced out by more dark rushing in to compensate. I have seen people on a spiritual path who have ended up with cancer because the emotional body was never addressed."

This felt right; this felt familiar. "So the emotional body which gives birth to the symbolism needs to be cleaned up in order for the physical body to reflect healing." I needed to sum up what he was saying in order to be sure I understood it.

"Yes. And so an emotion that's held for example in the colon, an old childhood wound that's not released, will result in disease. Because you can clean up the physical vehicle with organic foods and healthy eating, you can clean up the other vehicles with meditation and spiritual growth, but if you don't release that old emotional wound in the colon, it will intensify its darkness and erupt as cancer or other serious disease."

"So everything has to be cleaned up."

"Yes. Together. You don't want to take one or more vehicles too far afield on the highway without bringing the other three along. They have to be kept in relative alignment with each other."

I thought I understood what he was saying, at least on my level. No doubt it would mean more to me later, like all his teachings.

I was right. I had a shot at it a couple months ago. It was not until after my daughter lost her colon to ulcerative colitis, that she was able to understand the cause, and release the pain of being molested by her grandfather. Her healing came through a shamanic experience that brought her face to face with her dead grandfather and allowed her to feel love for him but also to express the pain. Symbolically, she was able to let go of the old "shit." I was honored to be with her at the time, sharing what I had learned—profoundly grateful that she "got it."

But to return to that afternoon in Alton's living room, I next asked him about part two of his therapy.

"What is it you are doing when you are laying on hands? Is it something you can't simplify into words?"

"Basically I start with a prayer that whatever unfolds, whatever is about to happen in terms of transformation, serves the highest for all concerned, and no harm to anyone. And then I put my hands somewhere on the person and enter a place where I am totally open to what is there.

"I may smell something, I may hear something, I may see something in a clairvoyant way. What I work with depends on what I experience.

"As an example, there's a fellow who arrived from California recently. He was at a birthday party I attended, and he had thrown out his first cervical vertebra. His head was about to explode.

"He got up on a table, and I just put my hands under his head so that the fingers were touching the first cervical vertebra, and I heard a sound, as on a pitch pipe. And then I heard a range of notes, but one note was missing. I'm not tonal, so I asked the birthday boy to bring a pitch pipe and run through the sounds until we caught the one that was missing.

"Everybody has thirteen sounds emanating from the body. If a sound is missing, a disease can be in place. 'In the beginning was the word ...'

"So when we found the missing sound, he played it over and over. It brought this guy into a cathartic release of a lot of old pain about never having had a father. The atlas, or first cervical vertebra is connected to the pineal/pituitary/hypothalamic system, which has to do with the crown chakra.

"In our perception at least the crown chakra has to do with the sky/father. His father was not there for him physically when he was little, so the atlas putting itself out of alignment was a way of bringing the person back to the issue of abandonment."

Continuing along the line of questioning about Alton's treatment methods, I asked, "When you see a client you give him a drink containing trace minerals. Why is that?"

"The Divine energy is grounded into the body through trace minerals. The other part is it gives a very nice clue as to the person's willingness to receive. It sets the stage, invites the person to receive. Here is some nourishment."

"Sure. You also ask people to remove any metal from their bodies. How does metal affect energy?"

Alton scooped Sunrise into his lap, where she curled up contentedly. "Much metal has a counter-clockwise rotation—and generally speaking, counter-clockwise rotation is into chaos. It's into the opposite of transformation. If metal crosses the mid-line, like the bridge of eyeglasses or a metal necklace, it confuses the mental body. It's very subtle. Sensitives can pick it up. In reality, it does affect everybody, although they do not notice it."

"So having it on your body when you are being worked on would be disruptive to the energy flow?"

"Yes, even twisting the hair in a bun could confuse the mental body. I knew a woman who couldn't make decisions. She came to me for help. Divine Mother told me to tell her to cut her hair and wear it straight. The woman got angry with me, for she had never cut her hair in her life. She went back to Oregon and continued her confusion. Some time later I heard she had her hair cut, and her confusion cleared up totally."

"How extraordinary! I guess you have to listen to those guides."

"Remember, everyone is absolutely unique. I wouldn't suggest that everyone who wears her hair up in a bun has issues with confusion; but for her it was right on."

I presumed it wasn't an issue for me, as my periods of confusion are mild and infrequent. At least I think they are. Anyway, my hair has been short and straight (except when it grew back curly after chemo) for the past twenty-five years. But then again, should the next pair of eyeglasses I get have plastic frames? Why not? Maybe that was silly. No. Why was I mentally bobbing to and fro? Maybe I have more mental confusion than I realize.

I shook my head and moved on. I had to. Approaching dusk was forcing me to give up the luxury of much diversionary thought.

"What is happening when you journey into what Michael Harner calls non-ordinary reality?"

"When a shaman works with a person, a shaman always travels. The shaman sends his or her spirit out from the body to travel into other realms to get whatever information is available for whatever transformation is to occur. That's a simplification. In the shamanic tradition there are three worlds, the upper world, the lower world and the middle world. The middle world is what we know as physical reality."

"Do you continue to take on the pain of your clients as you did originally with Lazara in Brazil?"

"No. It was a level of training that shamans go through, I guess. There are other levels, such as the belief that suffering is the only modality in which healing can occur. That is the Catholic paradigm. I was in that mode for a very long time, and had to sever my ties with the Shalom healing center in order to move out of it. It actually took years for me to shift through the paradigm and get through to where I could go."

Sunrise jumped off Alton's lap, arched her back high into the air in a luxurious stretch and padded off into the kitchen. I thought it must be a sign that it was time for me to pad off to Albuquerque. A couple hours had gone by as we talked. My head was spinning from so much thinking, my tapes had run into overtime; so I gathered my things, got a beautiful hug from Alton and left. His parting words resonated through my being: "It was good to be with you."

Yes, it was good to be with him. That's what it is all about. If it were not good to be with him I would not be feeling healthy and much lighter from all the garbage I had dumped into the great cosmic trash heap from the middle of his living room.

The thought made me chuckle as I drove the faithful old Subaru up to the main road, then turned left to descend into the city. Lights of Santa Fe were starting to twinkle in the dusk below. A faint fragrance of burning cedar—perfume of New Mexico—drifted into the car from adobe fireplaces warding off the late September evening chill. Bright red *ristras*, (strings of red chile peppers), hung from turquoise painted rafters and protruding ponderosa *vigas*.

Enchantment. New Mexico is the Land of Enchantment. Soon the luminarias would be lit as the Christmas season approached—lights to help the Christ Child find his way. Magic.

Soon too, pots of *posole* would be bubbling on the stoves. Housewives would be preparing traditional New Mexican tamales, spiced with rich red chile powdered from the *ristras*. In the pueblos, women would be grinding corn on sandstone *metates*, in the traditional way, for Christmas feasts and dances.

My mouth watered at the reminiscences of tamales and *posole* past. It made me meditate a little on the role of food in our lives. Far more than simple fuel for our bodies, food is companionship, love, family, nurturing, sharing. Food is energy, food is life.

As I traveled home that evening, I remembered many of the occasions in which food played a joyous part. Especially holiday gatherings, and oh yes, picnics! We must have had more picnics per year than any people I knew. Picnics in mountains, fields, by streams, even in our own back yard. You could write a history of my family by cataloguing the picnics we enjoyed!

Our life the past couple years had been no picnic, that's for sure—yet food still played an important part in healing throughout my journey back to wellness.

At the time when physicians had been working their medical marvels on me—and other healers had gently been prodding me into new ways of understanding myself, moving my blocked energy, and throwing out emotional garbage—Dr. Bob Downs had been there all along, supporting my three-dimensional body by making sure it received all the nutrients it needed.

On my transformational journey I had finally arrived in Albuquerque by way of Indian Country. I had traveled down old U.S. Route 66, made a left on Louisiana and a right on Montgomery, to Downs Nutrition Center and Chiropractic Clinic.

Here we are now in front of the building.

I am inviting you in.

Picnics by the Side of the Road

ROBERT M. DOWNS

The Nutritionist

If you enter the door on the right, you find yourself in a store stocked with vitamins, herbs, health foods, body building supplements and apparel. If you enter the door on the left, you find yourself in a chiropractic clinic waiting room. The Lady and the Tiger, only in this case there is no way you can lose.

Debbie is behind the desk. "Hi, Cynthia!" she smiles, glancing up from some paperwork. When I get my regular tests there, Debbie takes blood from my veins—but she's not a tiger.

Gayle, Bob Downs' wife, bounces out of the office. "See how nice your prints look framed?" She gestures at the waiting room wall, where two of my prints are now hanging. Gayle moves fast, but she's definitely a lady.

I agree they look terrific.

I am not here for one of my periodic consultations, but to pick up a printout on nutrition and cancer from a computer service to which Dr. Downs subscribes. This service gives him access to the very latest information in the world of nutritional research and clinical trials.

Debbie hands them to me. I go into the store next door to buy some vitamins, then take off for home. I do a lot of reflecting in my car. On the way I reflect back to how I found myself in that waiting room the first time.

We have a family joke that I must have starved to death in a previous lifetime—probably in a covered wagon heading west on the Santa Fe Trail—because my life journey finally got me from the east coast to the Southwest, my larder is always stocked to overflowing with home canned produce, and I never travel anywhere without provisions.

So it was entirely in keeping on this transformational journey that I had plenty of nourishment, both physical and spiritual, along the way. I call them my picnics by the side of the road.

Bearing in mind the astrologer's conviction that cancer is a metabolic disease, and aware that chemotherapy was playing havoc with my digestion, I began thinking that maybe I should find someone skilled in nutritional counseling to help me along.

As usual, as soon as I recognized a need, a teacher appeared. Yet another demonstration of the way the universe unfolds.

Doris Steider, one of my Layerist friends, took me aside at a gathering of artists at (yes, again!) Mary Carroll Nelson's house. Doris had been poisoned, as have many artists, by her art materials. She had also developed coronary artery blockage. Both problems had been resolved by nutrition, with the help of this chiropractor, Bob Downs. Would I be interested in having his telephone number?

You bet! Just the person I was looking for. I made an appointment.

After I announced myself to Michelle, the secretary, on my first visit, I sat down in a waiting room chair without looking behind me. Yikes! Every chair had a back support resting on it and mine had fallen over right where my tush was landing. Of course! This is a chiropractor's office! No wonder there were back rests on all the seats! I laughed at myself, thinking I must have looked like one of the Three Stooges. Michelle and the other patients waiting joined in. Any anxiety about meeting my new healer dissolved in the laughter.

Blushing a little, I settled down to consult a list of questions to ask Dr. Downs. Almost immediately a dapper, energetic, obviously intelligent gray-bearded man emerged from the hallway. He strode over to Michelle, who handed him my chart, walked over to me, transfixed me with piercing brown eyes, smiled, nodded his head in the direction of the hallway and in an authoritative voice invited me to follow him in.

On the way to his office I noticed a framed caricature of Dr. Downs holding a cornucopia filled with vegetables. As I settled into one of the two client chairs in his small consulting room, I asked him about it.

"Oh, yes, I had a phone-in nutritional talk show for years on an Albuquerque radio station. That write-up is from the newspaper. People would call in with questions and I would give them answers. It was a lot of fun."

I looked around. Two walls of the small room were entirely

obscured by authoritative looking books on nutrition. I mean the kind doctors would write. On a shelf above them sat a collection of antique medicine bottles.

He anted into the conversation. "I see you are going through chemotherapy."

"Yes, and I don't hear anything about nutrition at the Cancer Center."

"You won't!" His eyes glittered, warming to the subject. "Medical students have virtually no training in nutrition. As a matter of fact, doctors will discourage you from taking supplements unless there is an obvious deficiency. They will tell you to be careful, supplements can be toxic."

Hmmmm, this is one outspoken person. It might be fun to really get him going...

"Yes," I agreed, "one of the nurses told me, very earnestly and with great concern, not to take too many vitamins."

"Of course!" He laughed, raising his eyebrows and fixing me with an impish stare. "We have to educate them!

"But please understand I work with the medical establishment in the role of support, not competition. I work to keep patients in as good condition as possible, so they get through chemo without losing weight. If you lose weight, you lose strength. One of our goals is to maintain weight as best possible."

Dr. Downs' positive attitude was catching. I sat a little straighter in my chair.

"And all that most nutritionists will tell you is to go out and eat a lot of green beans!" He leaned forward in his chair.

I must have looked surprised, because he laughed, and went on to clarify.

"They don't take into account what is happening on a physical level from chemotherapy. First of all, when you have nausea, you can't eat."

Oh yes. For a certain period of days after each course of chemo I didn't want to eat any food except Ted's mashed potatoes. Mashed potatoes were just about all that would stay down.

"Secondly, if the lining of your digestive tract is affected by chemotherapeutic agents, how can you possibly assimilate all the nutrients that you do eat?"

That was a reasonable conclusion to draw. I nodded agreement.

"So logically," he carefully enunciated every word, "it stands to rea-son that you should eat food that can be easily digested, and power pack it with supplemental vitamins. Lots of complex carbohydrates. Pastas, rice, grains—this will help keep your weight up—

No problem. Pastas are one of my favorite foods.

"—and all the vegetables you can eat—

I love my veggies, too.

"—but cut out most fats—

OK so far; sounds a lot like the diet I have already adopted.

"—lean meat, chicken, fish in small amounts. If you eat too much meat and not enough complex carbohydrates, you lose weight.

Why didn't I realize that when I used to diet, and gain again, and diet again?

"No sugar—

OK, no sweat. Don't eat it anyway. Don't drink soda pop.

"—you can use olive oil or canola oil—

I love olive oil.

"—keep alcohol consumption to a minimum—

I gave that up when I learned I had cancer.

"—plenty of anti-oxidants, Vitamin C, E, beta carotene, leafy greens."

Yeah, this is sounding fine.

Dr. Downs wrote furiously on a sheet of paper and handed it to me. The paper was a prescription for vitamin supplements and other nutritional supports like digestive enzymes and acidophilus bacilli. He went down the list and explained what each supplement would do, end-ing the consultation with "Come back next week, fasting, for a blood test."

Somewhat dazed by the flood of information, I stumbled into the store next door and filled my prescriptions from the amply supplied shelves. I needed a lot of help. It's like looking for a specific spice in the spice section of a large supermarket. There's so much you can't see a thing.

To add to the confusion, most vitamins are produced by more than one manufacturer, so there are many choices. But Dr. Downs was very specific about which items and which brands he wanted me to take.

Yes, they are expensive. But even though I blanched at the total dol-lar amount, I remembered how much each course of chemotherapy costs. My first bill from the Cancer Center had just arrived, and I had been shocked. It made me very grateful for Ted's retirement insurance. It was many, many times the cost of vitamins.

The difference was that I was not insured for nutritional supplements. As far as I know, nobody is, which is regrettable.

When I got home Ted's jaw dropped at the sight of the bags full of bottles. "Are you going to move everything out of the kitchen cabinets?" he asked sarcastically.

"Sure, put all the canned goods out in the garage," I responded in kind.

"Can't they stuff all those into one pill?"

"Yes, they do have multiple vitamins and minerals, but this is a special program tailor-made for me."

He humphed out of the kitchen, but as time went on and he saw I kept my weight up and my energy level pretty good—despite the effects of chemo—he came to understand there was merit in all those little bottles. As a matter of fact, I have finally convinced him to take some basic support vitamins himself. This is more of an accomplishment than you might think. The Polish philosophy seems to be that enough vitamins are found in potatoes, sausages and sauerkraut.

The blood tests Doc Downs prescribed every six weeks or so provided a reference as to how nutrients were being utilized. He could then adjust the supplements as needed.

The entire subject of nutrition is just now coming into its own. Food is finally being seen for what it really is—the fuel that chemically interacts with body processes to provide all the nutrients a body needs to be in good working order. We call that health.

I can remember not so long ago when "health food" meant dry granola and plain tofu. Totally unappetizing, totally blah. Now most restaurants offer delicious vegetarian entrees.

Health food stores are no longer vitamin mills. They feature organic produce and wonderful substitutes for the old standards of cheese, meat and eggs. Also, people have broadened their tastes into international cuisine. Many healthful, vegetarian and low fat food items are now for sale that people never knew before. Like couscous and tabouli, tahini, baba ganoush and hummus.

This is not to say that everybody should become vegetarian. But it is true that people can find enjoyment in learning new ways of cooking. You don't have to sauté vegetables in oil, for instance; you can sauté them in a little water instead. I learned to use olive oil as a condiment rather than a cooking oil, because heating oils creates compounds that are not good for you. And when I am not actually using oils, I refrigerate them to avoid rancidity. Garbanzo flour makes delicious gravy instead of white flour. Briefly cooked veggies liquified in a food processor make wonderful soup. Spelt is a yummy whole grain you can cook like rice. There are lots of little tricks.

But you have to disregard some of the old ways of cooking, put effort into learning the new, and be open to different tastes and eating habits. I found, for example, that it was a mistake to try to make substitute foods taste like the real thing. You can't make a nut loaf taste like meat loaf, no matter how much ketchup you apply. It's doomed to failure. But you can enjoy the delicious taste of nut loaf in its own right.

The idea is to create new, appetizing, tasty dishes using fresh, wholesome low fat, unadulterated food, like oat patties, red lentil and ginger soup, Japanese soba with sesame seed dressing, a host of potato and pasta dishes, soups, salads, breads, stir frys. There's no end to the variety possible. Does that not sound more interesting than the same old tired meat and potatoes?

But this could be the subject of an entire book, so I'll leave that path and return to my own road to understanding.

In the evening, after that first visit to Bob Downs, I sat in my darkened studio, enjoying the mellow comfort of a fire warming my back. Ted had gone to bed. Sixteen-year-old Krutsch, the tabby cat purring in my lap, was the only other inhabitant of our home still awake. Little did she know she was to be my companion on a journey of awareness.

The night was brilliantly clear, as only a winter night in the high desert can be. My gaze penetrated the fire's reflections in the sliding glass door, moving to the piñon trees outside. They were bathed in a cascade of glorious silver light. The full moon hovering over Sandia Mountain was a magician. For surely, magic was afoot somewhere out there.

Shadows darted through piñon branches. Dead cherry tree leaves, levitating in some invisible breeze, flickered briefly in the moonlight before rearranging themselves under the piñons. The quiet evening had become filled with movement. Was it my imagination? I rubbed my eyes, wondering.

"No, this is a night the fairies and the devas are at play!"

Where did that voice come from? It was a gentle, feminine voice, unlike the accusing father voice I sometimes hear. She sounded like Pinocchio's good fairy.

I smiled and nodded, entranced by the magic outside my door.

Maybe they are there all the time, and we don't see them.

This time the voice in my head was my own. Or was it? It really did not seem to make much difference. I know there are other, unseen worlds out there, and sometimes it seems they interact with ours. How could it happen? Was it happening to me right then? The voice---I called her Intellect---kicked into our inner conversation.

"You know that all things, reduced to their most elemental, are nothing but vibrations."

"Yes," my self agreed.

"And you know human perception is limited to the vibrations within the range that our senses can pick up."

I agreed again.

"Well," continued Intellect, "Doesn't it follow that everything human beings perceive must also be within that range of vibrations?"

"You mean the trees, rocks, houses, moon, sky, people? Sure it makes sense. If they weren't within our range of perception we would not see them!" Where was Intellect heading with this one? I stirred the fading embers, giving them new life as flame.

"OK, you're with me so far. Let's go one step further. What if there are other existences with different vibrational levels from our own?"

"Well yes, my friend, I read that there are scientists at a government laboratory doing pure research on just that. They hypothesize there may be many different dimensions all occupying the same space."

"You're jumping ahead of me, Cynthia," Intellect gently chided. "Be patient. I want to take this step by step, so you really understand it.

"Pretend the alphabet is a bar graph, a linear scale, A to Z."

An image appeared in my mind:

A——F   G——L   M——-S   T——-Z

"Now, let's pretend we're on a stage. Let's say everything around us—trees, rocks, all the stage props, have a vibrational range of G—L. We have G—L vibrations also. That's why we can see the stage props.

"Imagine there are some other people who have the vibrational range of A—F. We can't see, hear, feel, taste or smell them because we are G—L. Their world of trees, rocks and people are all A—F, just like they are.

"Conjure up another group of people who are M—S, and so is the world they experience.

"And T—Z, same hypothesis. Are you still with me?"

Sometimes Intellect is impatient with me. But this wasn't too difficult so far. I nodded at Krutsch, who gazed back with those wise, glowing cat eyes that seem to see through space into eternity.

Intellect understood. "Now, all of us are on the same stage. We are all actors in our own little dramas, but we only see the vibrations that match ours, right?"

"Right."

"Suppose the T—Z people are on a T—Z train running across the stage. Maybe the A—F people are having a picnic in the middle of the stage. The train would run right through them and they would never know it. What do you think of that?"

"It's what the scientists are working on."

"I know, but I want to take this a little further."

"OK, I'm game."

"Take the case of Cynthia in our world, G—L. Let's call it the Blue World. She had a mastectomy and is undertaking a transformational journey to become well again. This Cynthia has a great fondness for dance and theatre.

"Imagine another Cynthia in A—F, —the Yellow world— who is a dancer. Could this possibly be another aspect of the Blue World Cynthia?"

Obviously, this was a rhetorical question. I stirred the embers again and settled down, facing the piñon trees, still listening, still open, waiting.

"Maybe another Cynthia in T—Z, —the Green World— is a renowned author. Could that be part of the reason the Blue World Cynthia decided to write a book about her experiences? Could this explain 'other lifetimes?' "

Why not? I was beginning to understand.

"And what if a person in G—L were a little different? Had a vibrational range of G—M, for instance? Wouldn't that result in an overlap of vibrational worlds? Could that explain psychic awareness in certain gifted individuals? A little bleed-through from the M—S world?"

Yes, of course it could.

"What do you say we call these vibrational worlds 'dimensions'?"

"OK by me." I liked the idea. Intellect was racing ahead now. I needed a moment to absorb. I held her at bay by getting up and going to the door, Krutsch in my arms. The shadows were still dancing in the moonlight. Who was out there?

I sent out a little prayer of love for all Beings. As I sat down again, gathering the cat onto my lap, Intellect resumed her teaching.

"The Huna of Hawaii believe that all lifetimes exist in the present moment, and you can access these other lifetimes in order to bring back information helpful in this existence."

This seemed to be almost exactly what Diane and Alton called the shamanic journey.

"But the movement between existences on the shamanic journey is not related to sensory perceptions. It is above and beyond and totally independent of our sensory apparatus. This is why the shaman must enter a state of altered consciousness to move in a different reality."

A-ha! It made sense. I don't know if it is "right," but it made sense. I remembered Dottee Mella exclaiming "My God! How simple! How simple!" when she finally understood the messages from that book of Kandinsky's writings.

I felt like yelling, "You're right! You're right! It's so simple!"

Instead, feeling lighter—is that what they mean by enlightenment?—and experiencing warm, deep contentment, I deposited Krutsch on the sofa, said goodnight to the devas and fairies playing in my back yard, closed the glass fireplace doors and joined my husband sleeping peacefully in bed.

Intellect was not yet through with me, however. As I was drifting off, she whispered in my ear, "Sleep well, my precious, but know there is more—much more."

CONVERSATION WITH DR. DOWNS

I always enjoy my visits with Bob Downs. As I suspected in our first meeting, it is easy to get him going! We have pursued just about every aspect of philosophical consideration on subjects from the economics of prescription drug marketing, to government policy, to how to live on a few acres of land.

This day, as I settled into my customary chair (have you ever noticed how we pick the same chair every time?) and pulled out notes and tape recorder, I promised to delete any political references that might be misconstrued. Bob laughed and said he would behave himself.

"Just how did you get into this career?" I asked. I think it is always interesting to learn the twists and turns of fate that bring people to where they are.

"When I was going to college, over twenty years ago," he began, "I was working for an exterminating company to help pay the bills. During my time there I was exposed to a rather substantial amount of chemicals. I became poisoned by the chemicals.

"I was hospitalized five days for tests. They did bone marrow taps, cut out two lymph glands and came up with a preliminary diagnosis of a virus of unknown etiology.

"I was so weak that I could not pick up a newborn child—my own. My lymph glands were so enlarged that I couldn't get my arms down to my sides. The initial workup implied that I might have early Hodgkin's disease or leukemia. There was very little delving into the possibility of poisoning.

"After three months I recovered to the point where I could return to work. Immediately on exposure to the chemicals I swelled up again. So it didn't take too much intelligence on my part to figure out there was a problem with contacting some very toxic chemicals."

His story reminded me of the Viet Nam veterans who had been exposed to Agent Orange. I shook my head in sympathy.

"While I was still recovering, there was an Osteopath/ Chiropractor in Kansas City who educated me on the subject of nutrition. He explained why I should build my body up from an immune system standpoint.

"That's probably the trigger that caused me to do what I am doing now. I was going to chiropractic college at the time, so I simply diverted my specialty from orthopedics towards the viewpoint of clinical nutrition.

"At the time, well over twenty years ago, nutrition was not in vogue—not even within my profession. We were looked at as either quacks or charlatans or oddballs. Of course that has thoroughly changed over the years, so that what we are doing now is quite accept-able."

"It's received some scientific credibility," I affirmed.

"Yes, it's achieved scientific credibility; although I should say the credibility was there then. It was just a matter of acceptance by the greater number of physicians. It sometimes takes years for anybody to accept anything different—"

"This is true." I was a little worried Dr. Downs would be off on one of his outspoken commentaries.

"—and it doesn't make something right or wrong. It just means it's accepted or not accepted."

He really was being good, just as he promised. I pushed on.

"What do you see as the relationship between nutrition and dis-ease?"

Dr. Downs rubbed his palms together, warming to the subject. "Logic says that God did not preordain people to become physicians so that they can take care of sick people."

Huh? What does he mean?

"The human body was designed, I feel, to function beautifully on that which the body was given for fuel. From a cellular standpoint it should be able to function quite adequately from birth until death with-out intervention. It is only when something goes into a state of mal-function that there needs to be intervention.

"So logic says: Food is fuel. The body is supposed to function nor-mally on that fuel. If it is fueled properly, it's going to function proper-ly with a properly working immune system and not require intervention."

Oh, I get it.

"But then we have to take into consideration genetics, chemical expo-sure, inadequacy of food matching the individual's needs, and the over- or under-supply of nutrients.

"The world knows now, for example, that you can get a form of car-diac myopathy from eating food grown on selenium deficient soil. That is well established. It is also well established that certain parts of the country have higher incidence of certain diseases than other diseases, depending on the nutrient content of the plants that are consumed.

"Excesses of nutrients can cause problems, just as deficiencies can cause problems.

"Again," he smiled impishly, slipping into ironic mode, "from a scientific standpoint humans with their intelligence like to feel they are the only ones who can make the determination as to what health really is.

"Health is a natural state of being! Disease is simply an abnormal state of being. If something malfunctions, it is up to the intervenor to try to determine what went wrong—to try to fix it." He paused, allowing me response.

"And you, as the intervenor, use your knowledge of nutrition to adjust the fuel, so to speak? Get the proper mixture to the carburetor?"

Dr. Downs grimaced at the simplistic analogy.

"There are three basic phases to thinking about human beings. You have to consider the spiritual, mental and emotional aspects as they relate to the physical.

"For example, it is well established that stress can cause various physical maladies. It affects the chemistry of the body, which can include the entire nutrient range of proteins, vitamins, amino acids, minerals, etc.—a whole package of things.

"And the physical aspect must also be considered, such as keeping the body in tune, in shape, well exercised, in order to function properly.

"So all three of those aspects have to be working in some degree of synch for a state of health to exist. We can exist sometimes without the benefit of one; but if you allow all three to diminish, you have serious problems."

"So anything that interrupts the natural balance..." I began.

"...will cause a state of disease." He finished.

"So as a nutritional therapist, how would you determine what is needed to bring the individual back into balance?"

"The first stage is—what's wrong? What body part seems to be malfunctioning? Then if you understand what usually makes that body part function properly, that's one part of the equation.

"Two, the evaluation of the mental and emotional state of the individual. Their background, where they come from, how strong they are, how weak they are.

"One eminent researcher on stress, for example, said there are three kinds of people. The first type of person is made out of steel. They can stand almost any stress or attack from anything and survive nicely.

"The second type of person is made out of plastic. You hit them hard and they get sick. They may fall down, but they will bounce back.

"The other kind of person is made out of fragile material, glass.

They break easily. We all know people who fit into these different categories.

"So that part has to be evaluated rather thoroughly, at least to get a feel for how much fight the individual has in him. There has been a lot of research showing that people who have a tremendous amount of fight in them have a higher degree of survival than those who just sit back and are accepting of their condition. That thesis, in my opinion, is very accurate."

I started to proceed to another question, but he had only paused to collect his thoughts. Before I could say anything, he continued:

"The other point is to look at the background or genetics of the person. It's been very well established that cultural preferences, the location of a person's birth and where their forbears come from also play a role in the genetic strength of the organism.

"For example, there are some cultures that never drink milk. If you expose them to milk, they will be unable to digest it. Other cultures cannot drink alcohol. Some cultures have never eaten beef; others don't even know what an orange is. Yet many of these cultures survive and live to a ripe old age without intervention. So you have to take into some degree of consideration where a person's roots originate."

I had heard of a tribe in Africa who live only on the milk and blood of their animals. Researchers who study them have to bring their own provisions, as they cannot survive on the same diet. It sort of illustrates a theory that newborn babies are rather like unformed lumps of clay, and that they learn to digest food from the act of having it fed to them.

"That would indicate to me that the process of learning to digest food is a stimulus/response," I ventured.

"It is a stimulus/response concept," he confirmed.

"From infancy, right?"

"From infancy," he reiterated, "and it goes back even generations beyond that.

"If Chinese people have never been exposed to cow's milk, for instance, how would you expect them to have the prearranged digestive patterns in their bodies to assimilate what they have never been exposed to for a thousand years?

"If people come from a long line of vegetarians, back generations, it would seem illogical to feed them an overabundance of animal protein, because their digestive systems wouldn't tolerate it."

"So when we are born we have a certain predetermined pattern?"

"Many experts seem to feel that way."

I was still seeking confirmation of my theory. "Then as we are fed as infants, do we develop new patterns?"

"The body is quite adaptable; however it is sometimes difficult to overcome thousands of years of genetics.

"I would point out, for example, a study published in *Nutrition Today* some years ago. They found that when Eskimos (whose diet in the cold country of their ancestry is odd by Western standards) move into our Western civilization and start consuming Western foods—de-vita-minized, high-fat, high-sugar foods—they developed all the diseases normally associated with Western civilization. It took about ten years. Tooth decay, gall bladder disease, colon and stomach problems, etc., etc., etc., which had been absent in their civilization before.

"Genetics also plays a part in the family history of some diseases. Why is it that in some families there is a tradition of females developing cancer when in other families it is unheard of? You have families where most of the members become diabetic. Why is that?"

He did not wait for a response.

"We can go on from disease to disease, finding family traits. Sickle cell anemia is another example. All those factors, our strengths and weaknesses, are what we are today, and that has to be given some consideration."

"Then, in addition, you use other, more definitive methods such as blood tests, right?"

"Yes. The next step after that thought process is to look at the clinical markers that have been established through the tests. In other words, the condition of the body chemically.

"Within that framework we find weaknesses that can be built up, by applying logic, scientific principles and knowledge. Areas that are already strong can be further strengthened. This will allow the organism to withstand the stress of whatever is attacking it."

This is a different approach from what I had thought. "So you are not healing by food—what you are doing is bringing balance back so the body can heal itself!"

"That's correct." He smiled at my obvious illumination.

"Dr. Downs, I have heard many times that we can get all the nutrition we need from our daily diet."

His face darkened as he spoke in clipped syllables. "That flies in the face of logic. It's good from a marketing standpoint, but it flies in the face of the logic of everything I have said up to this point—genetic strengths and weaknesses, cultural patterns, things like that.

"For instance, if it is true that everyone is the same—that we should all eat the basic food groups promoted by the various governing agencies regardless of culture and background, then nobody would be sick and everybody would be wonderfully well!

"There would be no people getting diabetes, eating the same foods as other people who never get diabetes. There are differences that have to be applied on a one-to-one basis to the individual who has the problem."

"My feeling," I added, "is that besides that, our food supply has been depleted of essential nutrients."

"In many cases that's true," he agreed. "Years ago, when we were in the white bread de-vitaminized, de-fibered era, the government supported the belief that was the correct thing to do. Then later on we found out that by taking out the vitamins, nutrients and the fibers, it was causing a problem. So they put them back in to feed this current generation. That will change again in the future. It is dependent upon profit.

"Something you are told is true now, may be found to be totally untrue and unscientific. In other words, the science of today may become the folklore of tomorrow, and the folklore of the past may become the science of today."

What an interesting thought! I gestured towards a century-old book of medicine on his shelf. "You just have to look at that old book to see how much medicine has changed. My husband has a similar book, in which the bad behavior of young girls in those days was blamed on reading novels and wearing store-bought shoes!

"But what about recent agricultural practices, pesticides, herbicides and the like? Don't they contaminate the earth's food supply?"

"Of course they contaminate the food supply. But to what degree is a subject of major disagreement in the scientific community. If you look at DDT, for example—did it cause problems, yes or no?"

"Yes, lots of problems."

"Was it banned, yes or no?"

"Yes, it was—none too soon."

"By the time it was banned, the multi-million dollar chemical companies had the capacity to produce new chemicals, which they could then test and prove are harmless for the short term.

"Then perhaps twenty years later they will be taken off the market, once they have been proven to cause harm to the environment. But then a new chemical will come along.

"The basic concept of using pesticides and herbicides to increase crop yield has nothing necessarily to do with quality of the food—only quantity, and profit to be gained."

I couldn't help but agree with him, bearing in mind one of my own frustrations with the government and the dairy industry.

There is too much milk on the market; therefore, milk prices fall. So why approve the use of the bovine growth hormone to make cows produce more milk? Then the dairy farmers must sell their extra milk cows for beef, which further drives down the price of beef. As a result, ranchers have to kill off their beef cattle to create an artificial scarcity to drive up the price again. And the small dairy farmers, unable to compete with the udderly superior cows (sorry, I couldn't resist that) are out of business. It just doesn't make sense to me—unless, as Dr. Downs suggests, the motive is profit by some organization who stands to make money from selling the hormone.

I was urging my clinical nutritionist on. "But people say we have a safer food supply because of the additives being put in food to preserve them."

"To some degree that might be true." He pointed to a magazine ad for breakfast cereal that was open on his desk. "From a marketing standpoint and the standpoint of shelf life! But again you have to remember that people who are paid to market a particular approach and interpret the data are going to do just that. They are going to preach a party line!"

Many were the times Bob Downs and I reorganized the government and the economic system during my visits to his office, and I enjoyed those conversations. But there were other patients waiting to see him after our interview. I was worried he was moving off into a political discussion, so I switched the track.

"I know you have a number of cancer patients that you help through chemotherapy and radiation. What do you do to support them?"

Dr. Downs laughed, aware of my tactics, and ran his fingers through his thick crown of gray hair. It matches his beard. "You have to consider that their bodies are already traumatized. Their bodies are being invaded, harmed and destroyed; certain organic systems are being challenged. We want to support all those systems in a manner that is reasonable and scientific.

"We also understand that radiation, even though essential, sometimes kills not only cancer cells but adjacent tissue. It damages the red cells, perhaps alters the white cells.

"Therefore anything we can do to provide nutritional support greater than the body usually would require, in order to build up the tissues so that they can withstand the stresses of the treatment, would be appropriate.

"The same thing with chemotherapy. Chemotherapy, though it is not the best of all things, sometimes is the only thing that will preserve life, based on current scientific knowledge.

"When chemotherapy is utilized, it causes damage to tissues. It causes nausea, and weakness, alterations in the red blood cells and white blood cells, and other body parts. Therefore, anything we can do to build up those tissues is important.

"So we simply look to the text books and ask ourselves, 'what helps to build up red blood cells? What helps to preserve them from oxidative damage? What helps to stimulate blood cell production?'

"We could even look to toxic levels of certain minerals: zinc, for example. An overage of zinc stimulates elevated white count. Would it not follow, then, that if you had low levels of white blood cells, giving zinc to the individual would cause the number of white cells to go up? Yes. It works.

"If a specific nutrient amount will cause an overkill, so to speak, a lesser amount will protect against damage caused by an outside factor.

"During chemotherapy and radiation, certainly there is a risk of pneumonia; there is a risk of malnutrition and weight loss because of nausea. Therefore, anything we can do to protect the body from nausea, and to stop any weight loss by providing caloric nutrients to the tissues will be helpful. Would it not follow that the body would be less apt to become ill from secondary problems and better survive the rigors of chemotherapy and radiation? That's our approach, and we have been very successful at it."

I nodded agreement.

"Again, I might add," he continued, "the idea is not to kill the cancer cells. I don't know how. We simply support the organism in its battle, by providing reserve troops necessary for the fight."

Dr. Downs finished talking, and looked at me inquisitively over his glasses to see if I felt he had fully answered my question. It seemed complete, so I moved into another area of personal interest.

"Do the long-term effects of chemotherapy interfere with absorption of essential vitamins and minerals from food?"

"In my opinion, yes," he responded, firmly. "That's why you have to supply these nutrients after treatment is finished, to keep things going. The damage does not go away.

"But remember, you are at a point where—if you cannot cut out a tumor or a node when they need to be cut out, and if you can't kill it with radiation or chemotherapy, and if you allow it to go on a rampage in the body and do nothing—you are going to die.

"Therefore, anything you can possibly do from a physical/chemical/spiritual/emotional standpoint to help the organism to fight the battle, that's what you have to do.

"And if the damage done by the agents of cure or control, such as surgery, radiation, chemotherapy, also cause peripheral damage, then you have to support the tissue the very best you can. In other words, you support the body while it is being attacked by the medical processes necessary to preserve life."

"What about herbs?" I asked, checking off another on my list of questions.

"Oh, absolutely! We should go back to some 'primitive' thinking of the naturopaths years ago. And we should also understand that, worldwide, perhaps ninety percent of the medications are from herbs.

"In the United States, it's only about twenty-five percent. We use the synthetic. We live in a market economy here, where herbs cannot be patented, so they are not profitable. Unless, of course, they are declared illegal, and a patentable drug made from them.

"I would point out that there are many herbs that are well-established in the literature as having cancer-killing properties.

"Mandrake, for example. One pharmaceutical company has certainly made millions of dollars with extract of mandrake.

"I would invite you to look at a major treatment for childhood leukemia, which is an extract of vinca rosa. Periwinkle.

"Look also at all the work being done currently on yew bark. You don't hear of a doctor prescribing yew bark, but you will hear of a chemical named fluordan, a drug from an herb.

"Many, many drugs and spices have anti-carcinogenic properties. More and more are becoming known." He gestured with his ball point pen. "And they will be developed.

"Many naturopaths have been familiar with mandrake and yew bark and others for years. I have never used them, because I don't have the clinical skills to manage a dangerous, toxic chemical."

Toxic? Herbs? "In what way are they dangerous, toxic chemicals? I thought herbs were much more benign. Herbs are natural, natural is harmless, right?"

Dr. Downs shook his head. "Some herbs are benign, other herbs are not. The fact that an herb is an herb, such as water hemlock, does not mean that nature has produced something that is good for you. It can kill a man in minutes."

"I remember the fellow up in the Jemez mountains who died from eating water hemlock a few years ago. He thought it was wild carrot."

"Right. One should be really careful in consuming wild plants. But it does not mean an herb is bad, either. Properly managed, in proper proportions, anything bad can become good, and anything good can become bad. Think of what two ounces of prune juice can do for you. But if you drank two quarts of prune juice, what would happen to you? There's good and bad in everything. A little sunlight is good for Vitamin D absorption. Too much, over a prolonged period of time, can lead to skin cancer.

"There is a large difference between herbs as grown in nature and highly concentrated 'drugs' made from the herbs. Sometimes pounds and pounds of herbs are used to make a tiny amount of concentrate. Then a highly trained medical professional should handle it."

"So the herbs," I summed up, "are best left to people who specialize—herbalists who have gained a great deal of knowledge from tradition, or previous experiments by other people."

"Of course. I use many herbs in my practice, but they are the ones I have a skill and expertise in using. And I stay within those guidelines."

In New Mexico we have an old Hispanic tradition of "curanderas"—women who, with their knowledge of herbs and wisdom, treat common ailments. Likewise, we have a large Native American population, whose medicine has traditionally depended upon herbs and ritual, performed by specially trained healers. Medicine men and women. Our more enlightened hospitals allow both medicine men and Western doctors to treat patients. It's a step in the right direction.

"Every culture must have a tradition of using what is available to it locally to treat disease. From these traditions, a lot of knowledge should be able to be extracted," I observed.

"Of course. Even today you will find that many pharmaceutical companies have teams in Amazon jungles and in darkest parts of Africa, looking for native remedies.

"We can easily reference the sixteenth century, when the 'witch doctors' in Central America were treating feverish conditions with the bark of a tree. Peruvian bark. When the conquerors came to Central America, and many of their troops were dying of this fever, they looked to see why the natives were not dying. From this observation came the remedy quinine."

And from willow bark came aspirin, I thought. Who knows what is yet undiscovered in nature?

"But quinine was not accepted in this country until the early 1900s. You see, all remedies have to withstand first, the test of time; and second, go through an acceptance level with professionals whose job it is to use the knowledge they have and shove aside any knowledge they do not have. That's called human nature."

He beamed invitingly, but I stirred uncomfortably, concerned that we might once again be close to slipping into a political discussion. Not that I mind airing our thoughts together. Many such discussions have brought me wisdom and awareness. But our time was nearly up, so I asked him the question I ask everyone:

"What do you think causes cancer?"

His answer was succinct and definitive: "I don't know!"

I laughed at his directness. Bob Downs is anything but indirect.

"Nobody knows, or we would not be working so hard to find out!" I retorted.

Dr. Downs leaned back and examined the ceiling, as if words were written there, then turned his full attention back to me. His speech took on augmented energy.

"Has it been shown that there is a genetic factor? Absolutely, in my opinion. Well, then, we have to think, does genetics cause cancer? Not all cancer, certainly, but there has to be a weakness there, which when confronted with exposure to a chemical, or situation that imbalances the human body, allows the cells to grow abnormally.

"A good example would be: hormone imbalances. If the body is rich in un-detoxified estrogen, can an estrogen imbalance in the body contribute to the formation of cancer in a susceptible individual? Yes.

"If a person on estrogen or birth control pills develops a cancerous tumor, do they put you on more estrogen, or do they take you off? They take you off estrogen, and then they give you an anti-estrogen drug, yes or no?"

"Y-yes," I stammered, taken off guard by his frontal attack. "Yes, they do," regaining my composure.

"Then is there a relationship between that cancer and estrogen? Logically, yes. It has nothing to do with marketing or right or wrong or who prescribed what.

"If, for example,"—his mounting emotion seemed to propel him forward— "you find certain pockets in the world where there is a high degree of esophageal cancer, and there is an imbalance in the soil of a particular nutrient, could one say that nutrient could have an impact? Such as selenium, for example. Yes! Does the research seem to indicate that bodies low in beta carotene and anti-oxidants have a predisposition to form cancer? The answer is yes! Are individuals who have less fiber in their diet more prone to cancer of the colon? Again, the answer is yes! Does it follow that people who eat cruciferous vegetables, for example, have less chance of cancer? Yes, because the indols and sulphur containing compounds within them have cancer-killing properties.

"All of these have been established through clinical trials. So you have to say there are so many variables as to the cause of cancer that to try to pinpoint a specific cause is next to impossible.

"But then, it brings you back to the original concept. If the organism is genetically strong, if the organism is fed the proper nutrient proportions for that particular organism, would that organism stand less of a chance of coming down with a cancer, or anything else, for that matter? The answer is definitely yes!"

What a good lawyer this man would have made! He pressed on, as if questioning a witness:

"Now, why do some people live to be a very ripe old age and never go to a doctor in their entire life, and simply die of old age? Why do other people develop very unique and odd diseases early in life with seemingly no explanation. Why?"

"Imbalance is the only thing I can think of," I answered timidly.

"They are not in synch with their environment—their individual, physiological environment. Their strengths and weaknesses are not in balance."

I was riding along the track with Doc Downs now. "Also their emotional environment?"

"Yes, that's the whole package. The three factors we talked about are critically important. All of these things need to be addressed. One is not necessarily equal to others. The greatest weakness receives the greatest attack."

That seemed to complete his answer. He settled back in his chair, waiting for the next question.

"What foods are definitely a no-no to eat?"

"Within the realm of nature, no food is a no-no. That sounds like an over-simplification. When the average person thinks of food, he does not necessarily think of a whole food, like the banana. He thinks of a banana-flavored thing. When we think of breakfast cereal we think of a packaged, grain-based product, not the grain itself.

"So within the realm of nature all grains, all vegetables, all fruits are perfectly acceptable from a genetic standpoint. If we ate nothing but whole foods, the problems resulting from de-vitaminized, de-fibered foods would never come up, would they? You would get it all, because nothing has been taken away."

He was logical, of course, to use his favorite word. But whole foods are not the basis of how we live. It only takes a field trip to any supermarket to see the percentage of whole foods as compared to gaily packaged, preserved, enriched, enhanced, sugared, colored, flavored, heavily advertised, top-of-the line junk. And unfortunately, a large percentage of this stuff is aimed at children. Kool Aid kids.

It gives me great pleasure to see mothers bring their children to our local co-op "healthy" food store, and treat them with fruit or frozen juice bars, while choosing from aisles full of organic fruits and vegetables, organic grains and wholesome (whole-some) foods.

In contrast, it pains me, knowing what I do now, to see baskets of soda pop, white bread, potato chips, snacks, high fat hamburger, cakes and cookies go through the checkout line. But the pressures of the media to buy these things are so strong, that we have complied, allowing our lack of understanding to be molded into desire.

Bringing my attention back to Dr. Downs, who was staring at me, eyebrows raised, as I lost myself in the supermarket, I asked how a person would locate a specialist in clinical nutrition.

"Being a clinical nutritionist is different from being a dietician. Dieticians do what they do, well. Basically, within the framework of my profession I am classified as a specialist in clinical nutrition."

"So could a person look up a clinical nutritionist in the phone book?"

"That's a place to start, but you find out very quickly, hopefully, the level of competence. The best way is the referral system. I believe in getting information from other people who have been successfully treated by that physician."

"One last question. Why do you think the rate of breast cancer is increasing so dramatically?"

"I think our environment is being chemically contaminated. I believe our stress levels are unbelievable in this country. Our level of satisfaction in life is low. I believe that the chemical components in our food chain have been altered, no longer meeting the genetic needs of the individual. I do think that our water supply is probably somewhat contaminated throughout the United States. As you combine all of these things, you then have a challenge to the system that is difficult to overcome. The body is simply going into a state of rebellion in response to this information.

"To cure cancer we need pure food, pure water and pure air. And to get them, truth needs to be told. There should be no restrictions on truth!"

As I put away my notes, Dr. Downs volunteered to get me the latest information on clinical trials of nutrients and cancer from the computer service connected with the University of New Mexico.

He did give me those materials. Although the reading was extra tough for anyone outside of medical academia to understand, I managed to plow through them to find, time after time, trial after trial, vitamins, minerals and anti-oxidants showed positive results, both in the laboratory and in real life.

The evidence is overwhelming. It just remains for the mainstream to accept this new information and use it.

As I leave Bob Downs' office, I always go home by way of

Albuquerque's North Valley. I travel up Rio Grande Boulevard, past luxurious homes and Arabian horse farms. The further north you go, the less luxurious the homes and less pedigreed the horses, until you emerge into open country.

The North Valley's fertile riverbed soil once supported a string of little villages, each built around its church, bordering a plaza. The city of Albuquerque gradually grew to engulf them, but the area has retained its agricultural flavor.

Busy streets lace through what once was empty countryside, but if you meander a block off of the thoroughfares you find yourself swept back two hundred years in time. Adobe walls enclose old Spanish-style farm houses. Aquecias, irrigation ditches, pass under roads and edge fields, bringing life to alfalfa and beans. Ancient cottonwoods provide welcome shade in summer and golden glory in the fall.

You may encounter some of those little village churches, still there, still ministering to people whose families have lived on that land since the conquistador Coronado came through early in the sixteenth century.

In this North Valley, tucked a block behind the busy intersection of Osuna and Fourth Street, a dirt parking lot serves the building in which Dr. Gary Moses, Naturopathic physician, uses all the arts of his profession, and a lot of creativity, to help restore people to health.

Gary's office is the last stop on my hypothetical journey from California to Albuquerque.

(My real journey, however is far from ended, for the journey of a soul seeking reunion with its Source goes on forever.)

Becoming Naturally Healthy
for Future Journeys

GARY L. MOSES

The Naturopath

Over his office door, a sign reads "Prevention Therapeutics." What it really ought to proclaim is: "Welcome to Gary Moses' Adventureland!"

"What?" you say, "a doctor's office is Adventureland?"

"Not an ordinary doctor," I reply. "A naturopath; and not an ordinary naturopath, either. On the other side of that door lurk amazing new adventures in therapy. Inside those offices, my acupuncture meridians were electromagnetically measured, sound waves passed through me, aromas stimulated my brain. My hair was analyzed, homeopathic medicines beefed up my immune system, and Chinese and Western herbs fortified me. My body was massaged, my aura cleansed, my brain balanced—and like a gourmet treat, I was baked, steamed, wrapped and kneaded!"

"Come on, Cynthia," you protest. "Who is this fellow, a magician?"

"No, just an unassuming but knowledgeable pixie with an irrepressible penchant for puns," I tell you, "like calling his local herb business the Garden of Eatin', or referring to himself as "Wholly Moses."

You groan at me, but I also hear you giggle. Laughter heals too.

My adventures in Mosesland began when friend Jami Morgan called me up one evening after I was back from the Virgin Islands.

"Cynthia, you have to see this man! He cured me overnight! Some kind of Chinese herbs...on Sunday, yet... I was so miserable. Yes, I'm fine. ...A wizard...nice as can be. ...Here's his number."

Her enthusiasm ignited mine. I telephoned first thing the next morning.

Dr. Moses answered, so low key I could hardly hear him. Sure, he could see me in a couple of days. We talked a few minutes about Jami's enthusiasm, made an appointment, said good-bye.

His earnest voice held the qualities of a child: deliberate, open. Impressions of the man behind the voice flowed through my head.

Children are in a constant state of wonderment, accepting everything as new information, without preconceptions...open...inventors think like children...must be an inventor.

This guy sounds creative...jumping mental barriers...leaping across accepted highways of thought into new pathways of possibilities...

The next day I had second thoughts about seeing him, but I wanted to learn more. Indecision. What would I be visiting him for? Was he like he sounded on the phone? The other healers were people whom I had contacted with specific intent. In this case, it seemed like I was moving from the specific to the very general. I had a lot of misgivings about becoming a patient of this unusual Doctor Moses.

What should I say to him? What mysterious things, after all, do naturopaths do?

Pretty much anything and everything, I later discovered, so long as natural forces and objects are their tools. In our own way, most of us practice some naturopathic therapies every day. They are natural and they have been around a long, long time.

Consider the Flintstones, for example. What do you suppose Fred Flintstone hollered when he stayed out in the sun too long?

"W-i-l-l-l-m-a!"

Of course. And Wilma probably went right out into the desert to pick some of that juicy aloe vera plant to soothe Fred's flaming nose. If Fred's knee ached from tripping over boulders, she might have filled a sabre tooth tiger bladder with hot water to ease the pain.

"Now Fred," she would most likely have said, "Keep that hot water bottle on your knee while you watch Pebbles."

Loving, though long-suffering wife that she was, Wilma no doubt would have rubbed Fred's shoulders when they hurt from lobbing his bowling ball half way down the alley. She would probably have slipped fresh dandelion leaves into his salad to help chase away the winter blahs. When he was crabby, she would have made him some nice, hot tea out of the little chamomile flowers growing by the doorstep, to soothe his jangled nerves. Fred must have needed a lot of tea! Wilma would have been an early naturopath.

But to return to what I was saying before rocketing off about Fred and Wilma, I felt a little ill at ease when I first entered Dr. Moses' office, because I had no specific focus.

His building seemed sort of unfocused too. The legendary Labyrinth of Crete crossed my mind. To the left, a consulting room. Straight ahead, a storage room filled with shelves of vitamins and Chinese herbs. Beyond the storage room, a hall leading to several treatment rooms, a bathroom and other halls. Offices of other practitioners opened off of those halls. One end of the building housed a natural foods restaurant.

I must have looked confused, because Rose, the morning secretary, led me by the hand past a wall covered with neatly packaged herbs, into the consulting room.

On the table was a small machine with an indicator. It looked like some sort of oscilloscope. Attached to it was an electrode and a probe.

Behind this apparatus, the bespectacled Wizard of Oz smiled welcome. Immediately, it felt appropriate to call him by his first name, for there was no pretense in his manner, simply artless concern, interest and welcome. Gently, Gary prompted my story, listening attentively, saying little, but making notes.

"Well," he finally offered, "maybe we should start by checking your meridians."

I nodded wisely, knowing about meridians from acupuncture. But how did he propose to check them?

Gary dipped the electrode in a little water and told me to hold it in one hand. With the probe he touched the thumb and fingers on the other, on each side of the nail. When he connected to the right spot, the little needle rose in an arc and the machine squealed a rising whine.

Next, he had me remove the shoe and sock on one foot. The procedure was repeated on my toes. While probing, he explained:

"Each of your organ systems relates to a specific meridian, which ends in points on the finger or toe. What we are doing is measuring the electrical resistance of the meridian, to see whether it is normal, or above or below normal.

"If it shows an abnormality, we can place a sample of a homeopathic remedy on top of the machine. The remedy then becomes part of the machine's magnetic field. If the indicator moves into the normal range, it is the correct remedy for that condition."

How clever! I thought. What a cool way to actually see how all those organs are working.

The thyroid registered low. He touched the probe to my neck. The machine whined, labored, but couldn't bring the needle to normal. Gary fumbled around in a case of little glass vials, selected one and placed it on top of the machine. This time the probe rose to acceptable levels.

"See how it works?" he beamed, as proud of the machine as if he had invented it.

He consulted my medical history. "I'm going to give you some homeopathic remedies. I see here you have plenty of nutritional support. I would only recommend you add Reishi mushrooms, which assist the immune system.

"There is another thing I might suggest, however, if you would like to become part of a research project."

Gary handed me a paperback book.

"Here is a book to read, called *The Cancer Cure That Worked.* It was written by investigative reporter Barry Lynes, about the work Royal Rife did, many years ago, with sound. Rife discovered that certain frequencies of sound would destroy cancer cells, and he cured a number of terminally ill patients. Unfortunately, his work was suppressed, but research goes on."

Pretty interesting news indeed. A cancer cure? I signed a release form to join the research study. Then I gathered up my reishi mushroom capsules, my homeopathic remedies (designed to stimulate the immune system, regress tumors and help out the thyroid) and drove home to read the book.

It was amazing. I couldn't put it down. I read through dinner and well into the night.

According to Lynes' book, in the 1920s Royal Rife built a series of microscopes that were the first to magnify cells so their inner workings could be studied—decades before the electron scanning microscope was invented. Rife's microscopes utilized quartz blocks and prisms to visually enlarge cells. The most sophisticated of his microscopes was two feet tall, weighed 200 pounds and had 5,682 parts.

Frustrated by the fact that staining slides killed the cells, Rife found that he could use polarized light instead of stains, enabling him to see inside living cells for the very first time.

In 1932, he also isolated the micro-organism that he believed causes cancer. Rife named it the "BX virus." He proved it was pleomorphic; that is, it could change form from a virus to a bacterium, depending upon its environment. He believed the BX virus itself did not cause cancer, but the virus' chemical constituents, acting on unbalanced cell metabolism of the human body, were what caused disease to manifest.

Rife found that, when exposed to a certain sound frequency, cells would blow up and be destroyed; so he invented a machine that could be tuned to certain frequencies, to kill various disease pathogens. Each pathogen was found to have a specific M.O.R. (Mortal Oscillatory Rate)—the precise frequency that would cause the cells to blow up and die.

In the summer of 1934, sixteen terminally ill patients with various kinds of malignancies were brought to his research facility near San Diego. After three months, fourteen of them were clinically cured.

Lynes' book relates that a number of physicians used the frequency machines very successfully for several years, until Morris Fishbein of the AMA tried to buy into Rife's enterprise. He was rebuffed. Subsequently, medical, cancer, pharmaceutical and political authorities systematically suppressed Rife's work. Unexplained tragedies occurred, including theft of an irreplaceable part of the microscope. One of Rife's supporters died under mysterious circumstances. Doctors who continued to use the machine lost their licenses.

In 1950, a man named John Crane met Royal Rife and worked with him to improve the frequency instruments by reinventing the design. Doctors in Salt Lake City began using the new machines but were forced to stop by the Salt Lake County Medical Board in 1958.

Crane was not able to get a patent until the machines were proven to be therapeutic, but he could not accumulate sufficient data to prove their effectiveness because physicians were not allowed to use them. He solved the catch-22 situation by leasing machines to people for research purposes only.

By 1960, ninety machines were leased for research, and an impressive data base of their therapeutic effectiveness had been compiled. Crane wrote and copyrighted a manual explaining the machine's use for research in various diseases.

Then his office was raided. Forty thousand dollars in machines and instruments were taken, along with all his records, private letters, tapes and electronic parts—all without a search warrant.

Doctors and private individuals were pressured to stop their research. Crane was put on trial in 1961 and sent to jail. Although he made many attempts to patent the machines after he was released from jail, he was never successful.

"Rife" machines are still being manufactured, but can be used only for research purposes. So OK, I was happy to be a guinea pig.

That first time, Gary sat me down in a comfortable recliner. Behind an orange gel, a light flooded the treatment room with warm softness. How can I describe that room? It was as complex as the Wizard himself. Its walls were lined with all kinds of interesting bottles, vials, books and exotic mementos. One corner held an old fashioned steam cabinet. The wall facing me supported a TV monitor, while another wall boasted two embroidered silk Chinese mandarin robes and hats.

"Those are for when I walk on people's backs," he smiled.

Was he kidding? I didn't think so.

My bare feet were placed on wet felt pads covering metal plates in plastic trays, connected by wires to a black machine about the size and shape of a large three-ring notebook. In my hands I held electrodes, covered, like the foot trays, with wet felt pads.

"This feels like an electric chair," I observed.

"Yes, shocking, isn't it?" Gary quipped back.

"You won't feel anything at first, because we are using high frequencies. You can hear them, though, if I route them through a speaker." To demonstrate, he spliced a tiny speaker to the wires and turned up the amplitude. A plaintive tone filled the room. As the dial tuned to a different frequency, the tone changed pitch.

"We use each frequency for four minutes, then move to another. As the frequency gets lower, you will begin to feel the sound vibrations. Any questions?"

"Yes. Why do you use different vibrations when only one affects cancer cells?"

"Because the others represent a tailor made program for you, that will enhance other body systems and destroy any pathogens lurking around."

"Oh. OK."

"Ready?"

"Go ahead, fry me." Gary turned the dials to 10,000 Khz, then moved the amplitude dial to full. I felt nothing. He turned to the wall, starting a videotape about cancer and the immune system.

"You should talk to your immune system," he said. It can hear you. Tell it nice things. Encourage it." He saturated a cotton pad with lovely smelling oil and taped it on my nose, dangling in front of my nostrils.

"Aromatherapy," he commented. "The brain likes it."

I was glad to know my brain and immune system were getting stuff they enjoy. Have fun, guys.

Every four minutes a timer went off, and Gary adjusted the frequency. The lower frequencies made my hands and feet tingle pleasantly.

I had a flash of how this might look to a person in the outside world. Here I sat, electrodes in hand, feet in pans, sound waves pulsing through me, having a conversation with my immune system, basking in orange light, watching television, with a cotton pad dangling from my nose. Come on, now! But at that moment it all seemed very fine and natural. After a few sessions, it began to feel like the most normal thing in the world. I kept those cotton pads in the car, so every time I drove, the aromatherapy worked again.

"God, what is that awful smell?" Ted wrinkled up his nose as he got in the car with me. One man's treasure, another man's garbage. Obviously, his brain works on different aromatics.

You remember those sexy perfume ads on TV around Christmas? I have often thought someone should make a perfume for women that smells like frying bacon. It would be the perfect fragrance. "Eau de Porque." Men would be attracted to it like flies to honey.

One day as I sat hooked up to the Rife machine, I asked Gary about the steam cabinet.

"Oh yes, that's a very nice, relaxing treatment. I put you in there for about ten minutes, then you rub an herbal liquid all over your body and I wrap you in elastic cotton bandages. While you sweat out toxins into the bandages, I massage your feet, do a little reflexology."

I thought that sounded really great. I had never been steamed, wrapped and reflexed. Next appointment, I had a new adventure.

It was delightful, except for the reflexology part. Having your feet rubbed is lovely, right? Not quite. It turns out there are places in your feet that send you into spasms of pain when pushed and prodded by expert fingers. The purpose of this prodding is to loosen up mineral crystals that form, interfering with proper energy flow to the organ systems reflexed by that particular spot. I did, however, leave that day feeling relaxed and refreshed, with a new appreciation of how a tamale must feel at the hands of those wonderful cooks who pat them, fill them, wrap and steam them to perfection.

Another day, another adventure. This time Gary hooked me up to a sound and light machine. In the goggles, lights flashed brilliantly at my closed eyes, while stuttering sounds crackled out of the earphones. Changing tempos and decibel levels bring the hemispheres of the brain into balance, I am told. It's a kind of psychedelic experience. You just have to give in and enjoy it, as the light and sound blot out all thought.

Having an empty mind is an unusual and curiously relaxing experience. How nice to give it a rest!

In addition to being a Doctor of Naturopathy, Gary Moses is a Licensed Massage Therapist, and a Doctor of Oriental Medicine. Gary also invents things and keeps bees. As a matter of fact there is not much that escapes Gary Moses' interest. His wonderful collection of original southwest oil paintings shares walls with "bee art," consisting of embroidery hoops decorated with dried flowers and weeds, filled with fantastic honeycomb shapes.

"How do you get them to do that?" I asked one day when I was attached to the Rife machine.

"You have to get inside their little heads and tell the bees what to do," he says. "You have to talk to them. Whisper in their little ears."

He must be kidding. He looks totally serious. I'm never quite sure whether he's joking or not.

The healing treatment I have come to most enjoy at Gary's hands (pardon the pun) is massage. Again, my cultural patterning insists that it may be all right for athletes who have sore muscles, but massage is entirely too suggestive for nice girls to enjoy. Best left to the intimacy of the bedroom. Nothing could be further from the truth.

Touch is our most basic need, after air, water, food and shelter. Research has shown that babies who are deprived of touch fail to thrive. It is the most ancient of healing techniques, and one of the most pleasant. To be touched not only relieves pain and muscle tension, but creates the same kind of feeling as when mommy took you on her lap, cradled and rocked you and made you think the world is a wonderful place. Euphoria. Why do so many people have difficulty allowing themselves to be touched?

We all carry stress as tension in our muscles. Relieve the muscle spasms, you release the tension and therefore the stress. Stress is not good for people, animals or geologic fault zones. When too much stress builds up, something breaks loose, or breaks down. Massage is a safe, pleasant way to relieve it.

Therapeutic massage, as opposed to sensual massage, is a skill which must be learned in an accredited setting. Therapeutic massage practitioners are professionals, licensed and certified.

I knew all that, but still felt a little nervous at the idea of lying naked on a table while some man moved his hands all over me! I should not have worried.

Helen, the afternoon secretary, led me into yet another room in Gary's maze of offices. She indicated where I should hang my clothes, placing a folded towel on one of the two massage tables.

"Lie down on your back and cover yourself with this," she indicated. "Enjoy."

She closed the door, leaving me alone. I hung up my clothes, climbed onto the massage table covered with a clean, white sheet and pulled the towel over me. Over in the corner, another orange gel diffused a fluorescent light. On a shelf, along with a tape player and tapes, were containers of various curious paraphernalia such as incense sticks, bottles of oils and rocks. Rocks? Yes, and a crock pot to heat them in.

He makes stone soup! I giggled, thinking of my granddaughter Emilie, whose kindergarten class made and ate stone soup flavored with barley, carrots, potatoes, celery and onions—and several nice clean river cobbles.

By the time Gary came in, I was relaxed, my head cradled in a round support, the towel covering me modestly from chest to knees. He dropped a cassette into the tape player. Soft, improvisational piano music drifted over us. A support form was slipped under my knees. Gary selected a bottle of oil from the shelf, warmed it in his hands and lifted my right arm, the mastectomy side, straight up, gently rubbing the fragrant oil into my hand. It felt wonderful.

I snuck a glance at him. Eyes closed and head bowed as if in meditation or prayer, he began rubbing the muscles of my arm down towards the shoulder. It felt good, soothing, until he came upon a spot near my elbow that must have sent him a signal, because he pressed it hard with his thumb. I squirmed in discomfort.

"That needed some attention," he blinked, totally present now, massaging the attached muscle up to my shoulder. "There, that's better." Yes, it was. The arm fell limply to my side.

A comparison with the radiation therapy table came to mind. No question, this was more comfortable! Soft lights rather than bright lights; nurturing human touch in place of a big buzzing machine; relaxation as opposed to tension; focus on wellness instead of focus on disease. They may both be effective treatments. But as for which I prefer to undergo, massage wins (pardon the pun again—it's all Gary's fault) hands down.

Gary's strong fingers massaged my always sore right shoulder, moving to the back of the neck, base of the skull, ears, other shoulder and arm; meanwhile keeping up a stream of conversation about the life of bees. As he stroked my forehead and rubbed my sinuses I learned how the queen bee develops. As he worked on each of my legs in turn I heard about bee mating flights, honeycomb building, flight patterns and bee dancing.

Gary brought another towel, placed it over my hips, moved the first towel up to uncover my belly and began to massage my stomach. Lunch kind of gurgled around as his probing finger tips stimulated all those intestinal organs.

"Oh, there's an avocado sandwich!" he chuckled, "and there's an apple over here!"

"No, miso soup and salad," I corrected. "No apple."

"Now turn over," he directed, holding a towel above me to protect my privacy.

Privacy wasn't the issue by then—energy was. I felt as limp as wet spaghetti. Forcing my muscles to turn over brought me back from drifting along with the bees. Somehow I managed to flop onto my side and plop down on my stomach, exhausted by the effort.

Gary draped the towel over my rear end, moved the support underneath my ankles, and began to work on my feet. He must have gotten rid of those crystals during reflexology, because this time it did not hurt.

"How do you know what areas need special attention?" I asked.

"I can see the energy."

"You can actually see it?"

"Yes. I can see how it flows."

"Can you see auras, too?"

"Sure. Yours is blue and yellow."

"Neat! I always wondered what color it was." I had been reading Barbara Ann Brennan's book *Hands of Light*, which has beautiful color paintings of auras and energy flow. I really believed Gary could see it; I only wished I could too.

I have been practicing. I look at my hands in dim light and check my image in the dark mirror when I get up at night to go to the bathroom. There's just enough ambient light to illuminate bluish haze and wisps of color around my silhouette—or is it my imagination? I sigh, wondering, and go back to bed.

Gary lifted my ankle and ran his fingers along the side of my shin. It was a hurt that felt good. Up the side of my thigh *(ouch)* to the hip that had been painful; he dug around pretty hard there. The other leg got the same treatment, then he began to massage my back.

Abruptly, he pinched the skin between his fingers and pulled it hard, away from my backbone.

"Hey! That hurts!"

No response, just another pinch and pull higher up. Quickly, before I could do anything but yelp, he yanked another, and another, travelling up my backbone.

"Gary, why did you do that? It hurt a lot!"

"You had adhesions. I pulled them loose."

"Jeez, I hope I don't have any more." His hands were smoothing my back muscles now, lulling me into relaxation again.

He moved on to my sore shoulder, pulled my arm behind my back and massaged the muscles around the shoulder blade. Then he walked around to the front of my head, pulling the whole arm forward, hard, stretching it out. It hurt. The Reach to Recovery lady was right. I will have to stretch that arm forever! The other arm got stretched too, but there was no pain.

When I was all stretched out, totally relaxed, he put another towel on my back, rubbed it comfortingly, then ran his hands from head to toe, about six inches from my body. He put one hand on my head and one on the base of my spine.

"What's that for?"

"I'm balancing your aura. People don't realize when they come for massage, they get their auras balanced too."

Another pat on the back. "Take your time. I'll see you outside."

I lay there for a minute or two, just experiencing how my body felt. Warm, tingling, relaxed. I hated to get up. Putting on my panties, the knees moved easier. Pulling on my blouse, the arms moved more freely. I felt lighter, especially through the shoulders, like a big load had been taken off my back.

In the outer office, I couldn't resist giving Gary a big hug. He looked surprised, a little embarrassed, but laughed at my blissful expression.

"Everybody looks like that coming out of there," smiled Helen.

Driving home, I noticed it was easier to turn my head and body to see traffic around me. My sore hip didn't hurt any more.

Oh, how easily one can become addicted to what feels good! I guess the trick is to find feel-good things that don't mess up the body or mind, and are legal. Massage is one of them. Most of my subsequent visits to Gary were for massages.

Those visits vary according to what is bothering me. Sometimes Gary puts ice or heat on sore spots. Once he put on hot rocks. Now I realized what those stones were for. And once, when I had developed a persistent sciatica, he actually massaged the pain from my back, chasing it through the hip, down the outer side of the leg and out the ankle. The pain was gone!

"That was one of my finer moments," Gary admits, modestly.

I see him now in the same way I used to see a family doctor. I bring him my sinus headaches, my sore muscles, my flu, my arthritic thumb or sprained wrist.

He gives me custom-ground Chinese herbal tea remedies, homeopathic medicines, special vitamins and herbs, comforting lotions, massages and new thoughts. A whole lot of new thoughts.

Once I asked him how he would describe himself. I was getting ready to write this chapter, and finding it hard to fit him into any specific category. Gary thought a couple moments, then offered in a gentle voice, "How about Love?"

Yes, that fits. And it is the best of medicines.

Although much of Gary Moses' knowledge evolved from his own boundless creative curiosity and interest in all living things, his credentials are derived from accredited institutions here and abroad.

As a massage therapist, Moses is a diplomate of the Anderson School of Scientific Massage in Princeton, Illinois. He earned certification as a Doctor of Naturopathy at the Anglo-American School of Drugless Therapy in England. His Doctorate of Oriental Medicine came from the International Institute of Chinese Medicine in Santa Fe. Gary also spent considerable time in China studying Chinese medicine and healing techniques.

Over many years he attended classes and seminars in herbology and related subjects, constantly adding to and updating his scope of knowledge. He just never stops learning—wouldn't stop, even if he could!

Gary the inventor has created many interesting products, such as a meditation chair, which beams colored light at clients, while playing relaxing music and blowing therapeutic aromas up from below. Also seed sprouting kits, new herbal products, tea bags on a stick—you name it.

At the consultation table, on the day of our interview, the little oscilloscope machine between us, I opened the conversation with the same question I always ask: "How did you come to do the work you do?"

Gary's eyes lit up.

"When I was younger, my dad had a honey company with about 1500 hives of bees. We would deliver honey to health food stores, and while we waited for the paper work to be completed, I would check out the books about massage, herbs and nutrition. I always was interested in plants and flowers, so over time I took courses in herbology, acupuncture and the like.

"Then one day when my dad was working with the hives in southern New Mexico, next to some Bureau of Land Management land, he got sprayed with Agent Orange left over from the Vietnam war. The BLM was trying to eradicate salt cedar bushes that were using up too much water."

"Agent Orange?" I was incredulous.

"Yes, and the next morning my dad was in convulsions. We had to take him to the hospital. The doctors did not know what was wrong with him. He was in the Veteran's Hospital for about three months.

"Even after he got out of the hospital, he was really pathetic. He was on a lot of drugs, but still was non-functional. I told my mom I did not think all those drugs were the answer.

" 'There has to be something else,' I said to her. I had been reading a lot about vitamins, so I suggested we give him vitamin C and other supplements. Soon he started feeling better.

"Up until then he thought vitamins were for health fanatics, weirdos and little old ladies; but when he saw how much they helped him get well again, he bought a little convenience store and began putting in a stock of vitamins and getting rid of the candy and cigarettes. I set up a massage table in the back, sort of like a hobby.

"That was over sixteen years ago. People responded to the health food store amazingly well. My parents had to move out of that little store and into a bigger one. It's been a going concern ever since."

Moses Kountry Health Food Store was the place where I found my Jason Winters' Tea, back when this whole breast cancer thing started. Funny how the web of threads connect.

Gary paused while I commented on the connection. He nodded wisely, resuming the narrative.

"My father's health just continued to improve. He's seventy-four years old right now.

"Meanwhile we had to sell the bee business because the interest rate skyrocketed to twenty-five percent and we couldn't borrow enough money to maintain our inventory. After we sold the business, I had no source of income.

"Well, I figured, I still had my two hands, so I put an ad in the paper, went around to health spas doing massages and set up an office in the garage at my home. After a while my wife got fed up with having so many people trekking through our home, so I moved my little business into the building my parents had vacated.

"Speaking of connections," he continued, "because Dr. Zeng from Santa Fe needed a place to have weekend classes in Albuquerque, I told him I would trade a room at my place for classes in his acupuncture school. That's how I got started in acupuncture, and from there I moved into Oriental medicine and study in China.

"A fellow who used to bring herbs to my parents' store wanted to sell his business, so I bought it by paying him a little every month. That's how I started in the herb business.

"That building I was in started to deteriorate, and the landlord did not want to put any money into it, so we remodeled this building, and here I am!" Big smile.

I returned the smile, refraining from comparing the building's designer with the Minotaur. Instead of that, I moved into the meat of our conversation about naturopathy.

"Tell me, Gary, what naturopathic physicians really are. How do they work?"

Smoothing his hand over polished forehead and thinning hair, he responded earnestly:

"They work with nature, and they recognize plants and other natural objects as having an influence on people. In naturopathy we don't try to diagnose disease, we look at the character of the problem. We don't treat the disease, we treat the nature of the condition.

"If a person comes in with a hot condition like inflammation, we use herbs that have a cool effect. If someone comes in with chills, swelling or poor circulation, we wouldn't recommend things that are cold to eat. Cucumbers, watermelon, adzuki beans or mung bean sprouts have a cool nature."

"That's kind of like the acupuncture theory of yin and yang, isn't it?"

"Yes. If a person has a heat condition we recommend cold; or if a person is dry, we recommend nutrition and herbs that are moistening.

"We work on people with natural things. We recognize the relationship of people to food and our environment. We use hydrotherapy, massage, various massage liniments, music, aromas. We use different colors of light. There are certain colors that affect people subconsciously. Blue is calming; red is invigorating; green can be calming as well; yellow might help with digestion.

"Colors have a relationship to the time of year, too. In winter it's darker colors; summer's colors are lighter. In the fall, it's the harvest color group; in the spring, it's the new growth, greens. Those are the colors we relate to seasonally."

Gary paused to remove a pen from the pocket of his lab coat.

"Anyway, the main thing with naturopathy is that we recognize human beings have certain natures, and we work on strengthening people so they can resist pathogenic factors." He placed the pen neatly beside a pile of papers and looked back at me.

"OK" I agreed, "So you are strengthening the whole person."

"Yes. Naturopathy is really based on tradition, as is Chinese medicine. It is based on thousands and thousands of years of experience, where they have found out certain things that have helped, and other things that have to be avoided."

"Is naturopathy an English tradition?"

"English and European." He gestured towards the wall of herbs outside the door. "In New Mexico we have a four-hundred-year-old tradition of naturopathy. Spanish people brought herbs from Spain and Mexico. *Curanderos* and *curanderas* in New Mexico use herbs. They use nature.

"Naturopaths have expertise in working with degenerative, chronic disorders, which require a long period of nutritional support. I don't work on broken bones or that sort of thing, where people have to go to a hospital for x-rays or surgery."

"Regarding cancer, is cancer hot or cold?" I asked. I was curious, because the astrological counselor had recommended warming foods and spices.

"That would be like a degenerative, chronic, cold stagnation," he answered, peering over his glasses at me. "A tumor, in Chinese medicine, is considered to be a kind of stagnation of the blood."

Cancer is stagnation! What symbolism here! Stagnation of the blood, stagnation of the life force, stagnation of desires and following one's bliss, stagnation of emotions, fulminating deep within our bodies.

Gary reached over and touched my arm, eyebrows arched in question.

"Oh. Yes," I stumbled, coming back to the conversation. "What are the techniques you use as a naturopathic physician? I know you use homeopathy. Perhaps that would be a good place to start. What does homeopathy do?"

"Homeopathy uses natural substances like minerals and herbs in very minute amounts to stimulate the body. Some herbs are known to be toxic—like poison ivy, for example.

"A long time ago, a certain Dr. Hannemann in Germany found that if he took the toxin, diluted it and administered it to a patient, the original symptoms caused by the toxin would disappear. The diluted toxin would activate the body to heal."

This concept felt familiar.

"It must be similar to anti-allergy shots, where people allergic to dog dander, for instance, are injected with tiny amounts of it over a long period of time to increase their tolerance."

"Right," he confirmed. "That's essentially the same thing. It's like taking a vaccine. Homeo means 'the same.' Homeopathy uses the same thing that caused the disease to alleviate the symptoms. But you are using it to stimulate the body so that the body can heal itself."

"I presume this is a more long-term, gentle approach than giving a drug."

"Yes," he nodded, folding his hands on the table, leaning forward as if to make sure I understood. "Homeopathy in this country is recognized as being non-toxic, and is sold over the counter. The medicines have no side effects, because it's in such small amounts. In fact, in some medicines, there is nothing left in the remedy except the vibrational pattern. It's based on the fact that water has memory."

That was news to me. "Water has memory?" Gary didn't pause.

"Some of the solutions have been diluted 500 times. One milliliter of a substance will be diluted with ten milliliters of water. That's called a one-X or one dilution.

"Then they take one milliliter of that solution and add it to ten milliliters of water. That's called a two-X dilution. If they do it 500 times, the end result has nothing left in there—just the vibrational pattern of what existed before.

"But that vibrational pattern is enough to create change.

"If people are really sensitive to something, the sensitivity can affect them mentally. Take odors, for instance. Someone could have a kind of hysteria provoked by odors. Psychological counseling is not going to change the biochemistry of the individual to neutralize the sensitivity. There are some homeopathic remedies that will actually effect change, rather than just having people learn to cope with it."

"But homeopathy works for demonstrable physical ailments as well as emotional ones," I interjected.

"In fact," he observed smiling gently, "it's really difficult to know when the mind stops and the body begins. A lot of times the threshold of going from one to the other is very, very subtle."

We talked for quite a while about mind-body relationships, plunging into detail about various cases, and rocketing off into worlds of spiritual speculation. During one energetic gesture, I knocked the electrode connected to his little assessment machine off the table.

"I've noticed you have a very interesting machine here," I remarked wryly, bending to pick it up. "Could you tell me what it's called and how it works?"

Gary did not pick up on my sarcasm, remaining earnest.

"This is a real simple machine that was developed in Germany. It is a continuity tester that measures the electrical resistance going through distal acupuncture points located on the fingers and toes. In physics, this instrument is known as a wheatstone bridge. There is a meter, and a magnet. When the instrument is turned on there's a force field around the magnet. You can put a sample of an herb or a mineral on it and learn if that sample is compatible with your body chemistry. Right now these instruments are used a lot in dentistry to see if people are sensitive to different amalgams."

"Can it measure anything for its electrical resistance?"

"Yes."

"Anything in nature? Like you could put a rock on there..."

"...and find out if you are compatible with that rock."

"Neat. I believe it is based on the assumption that each of the body's systems has a termination point on the fingers and toes?"

"Right. In fact, that's why we have fingernails. A lot of people don't realize that."

"It never occurred to me to wonder why we have fingernails!"

"The fingernails and toenails are dielectric. The nail itself regulates nerve energy. The material in the fingernail controls movement of electricity in the body to keep it balanced."

Amazing. Can you imagine how much more we don't know about the workings of our bodies? The fact that we live, breathe, eat, digest, heal, sleep, grow—all without conscious effort—is breathtaking. Even our fingernails serve biological functions. You have to be impressed by the Designer.

I wanted Gary to explain some of the other methods of therapy he uses, since some of them may be unusual or unknown to the majority of people.

"How about talking about reflexology, Gary?"

He pushed back his chair, tapped my knee and watched my foot jerk upwards. "That's a reflex!" he chuckled as he saw the surprise on my face. "That smile is a reflex too! Reflexology is based on the idea that there is an internal and external relationship. It is derived from observation and experience maybe—who knows?— 10,000 years ago.

"Someone would have a stomach ache and it would be noticed there was another place on their body that hurt, which, if it was warmed or massaged, would cause the stomach ache to get better. Over thousands of years they developed a system of points that relate to internal conditions. So by massaging a point on the feet we are influencing the function of some internal organ."

"Why is it always done on the feet?"

"It isn't, necessarily. It could be done anywhere on the body. It's just done on the feet because that is a place where people are more sensitive."

This sounded like it had a lot in common with acupuncture. "Are these the same points acupuncture uses?"

"Yes, because a lot of points acupuncturists use are just places that are tender. They are called ashee points. That's where when you push on it the person goes *aaahhh!* —"

"Sheee! Gary, stop it. This is just too corny."

"OK, ahiee! points. Is that better? Anyway, to give you an example, there was a lady whose seat belt in an accident caused her stomach to go into spasm. She was unable to evacuate, and her abdomen became dangerously bloated. The usual medicines didn't help. All I did was dig around a really sore spot on her foot in the area that relates to the small intestine. The next day they called me to tell me that just after I left, the blockage was released and her elimination returned to normal. In spades."

"So rubbing that spot released the spasm?"

"It was a nerve reflex that released the spasm."

"These acupressure points, then, are not necessarily nerves?"

"They are part of the sympathetic nervous system."

I thought of Gray's Anatomy, which I had studied in art class. "When I think of the nervous system, I imagine diagrams that look like trees."

"That's the central nervous system. This is part of the autonomic, or sympathetic nervous system. It makes our heart beat, our liver work, our digestion work, all automatically. It's commonly known in traditional medicine that there are external places where internal problems are manifested. Like soreness in a certain part of the body might mean kidney disease. That's pretty well established.

"But we are not using that knowledge just to diagnose the person, we are using it to treat the person, as a therapy—to massage an area as a reflex. You see, in many cases you don't want to work directly on the area in trouble. I wouldn't have wanted to work on that lady's stomach, because it might have made it even worse. But if I work someplace else that is a reflex of that organ, I can release the tension, get that energy moving."

"Is this what massage does as well?"

"Right. A lot of people say they want a massage because it is pleasurable and makes them feel better; but in fact, the tension they carry in their muscles affects the function of their internal organs.

"There's a psychologist, Dr. Ida Rolf, who recognized very dramatically that certain psychological processes would manifest in physical changes. She found that self image and self esteem were reflected in body posture, so she worked on people by stretching connective tissue—hard, with her elbow. During that process, people would unload some of their repressed emotions. That was a healing process. The process became known as Rolfing."

I had heard that Rolfing hurt. No wonder people let go of their repressed emotions.

"If someone were hurting me I would let go of a lot," I observed. "I think I would yell and scream and be bloody angry."

Gary took off his glasses, rubbing his eyes. "Uh huh, but it's not as simple as that. You do one layer at a time, like peeling an onion."

That onion metaphor again! There must be something to it.

"You do one layer at a time. When you're pulling and stretching it allows people to be objective about what they were suppressing before. Getting rid of the next layer allows things that are more deeply buried to be exposed and dealt with. You see, when certain situations happened at different times in their lives, they did not know how to deal with them, so they carry them around in the body. And that manifests in physical posture."

"And disease?"

"Yes, of course."

Here again, in different words, was what Dottee Mella had first told me, as well as Diane Polasky and Alton Christensen. And it was, as I progressed along my journey, one of the things I learned about myself. I had carried around a heavier load than I realized.

That train of thought was too profound to explore in our allotted time. Other patients had scheduled appointments, so I felt I should keep focused on therapies naturopaths employ.

"Iridology is another technique you use. Would you please tell me about that?"

"Iridology is part of naturopathy, and again, it goes way back. A long time ago in Europe a young man named Ignatz Von Peczely noticed that an owl that had broken its wing had a separation in the iris of the eye. As the wing healed, he saw that the eye knitted back together.

"At that time there was a war going on. He was working in a hospital, so he began keeping track of the relationship of soldiers' injuries to the iris of their eyes. Using that information, he developed the first chart showing the relationship of different parts of the body to different parts of the iris.

"In the United States, Dr. Bernard Jensen built upon Peczely's work, taking photographs of hundreds of thousands of patients' eyes and the case histories related to them."

Gary turned to one of the bookshelves and pulled out a large, thick book. He opened it to beautiful full page color photographs.

"This reference book has color plates showing some of these points. In iridology, we can recognize different stages of disease, all the way from acute sensitivity with minimum degeneration to life-threatening illness. It is mapped on the iris. It shows in the quality of the eye's texture and little lesions which occur there.

"I have a camera to photograph the eyes. I compare the photograph to these charts. We have to take into consideration the rest of the person; emotions, stresses, toxic exposure, etc. It's really one more non-invasive diagnostic tool. Many times we see a pattern that may lead to illness and we can change that with appropriate herbs and nutritional support. The eye will reflect the progress to better health."

Helen's voice could be heard greeting another patient at the front desk. I scanned my list of questions to find we still had not covered many of his interesting procedures. Sitting forward and speaking more rapidly, I asked Gary about other diagnostic tools, such as hair analysis and blood work, hoping to "get a wrap" in a few moments.

But Gary was not to be hurried. "We can and do use blood tests, but remember, I am not looking for diseases. I am looking at how things are functioning. If the person has a serious problem which requires intervention, I might suggest they see a regular doctor. Some people come to see me that really should be in a hospital. They are out of control, they have lost the ability to help themselves. I'm not really set up to handle cases like that.

"If it shows on a blood test that they are low in iron, for instance, of course I could give them herbs that have iron in them. Tonifying, strengthening herbs. Or if it shows they have fluid retention, we can give them herbs to help that—or if they have a problem with their blood sugar, I can talk to them about their diet. I could tell them what foods contribute to the problem and recommend that they eat small meals more frequently, so their blood sugar level remains more stable."

This sounded a lot like the real name of Gary's business, "Prevention Therapeutics." I wondered aloud how many diseases could be prevented without the use of drugs. All drugs, I knew, have side effects.

"I should think there would be a lot of chronic conditions that are usually treated by drugs that could be treated more naturally, like high blood pressure, for instance," I ventured.

"With high blood pressure we recognize the psychological components, like when people repress resentment. There are many factors that can influence blood pressure, such as water retention, frustration with career or life situation, or just clogged arteries. Absolutely, diet has a lot to do with that, and more and more doctors are recognizing it."

Helen came quietly to the door.

"I'm sorry, Gary," I apologized, "but I'm afraid we'll need more time to finish this conversation."

"You have an appointment for a massage next week. Why don't you bring the tape recorder and we'll talk while you are getting your massage?"

A novel thought: an interview punctuated with thumps, groans, yelps, and sighs of relief and pleasure. It might sound pretty strange. But I agreed, grabbed my stuff, thanked Gary and waved good-bye, brushing past an elderly woman conversing briskly in Spanish with Helen as she was led into Gary's office, cane in hand.

A week later, I was lying on the massage table under my towel when Gary entered.

"How do you start this tape recorder?" he asked. I told him. He pushed the button, set the machine on the other massage table and began arranging his paraphernalia. Grabbing my ankles, pulling the legs straight, he estimated the difference in their length. Then he took two wedges, and placed them under me.

"I put these wedges under your hips to offset the difference in your legs' length. I put one higher, to relax the connective tissue. On the leg that's shorter, I put it down lower. The way your body presses down on the wedges stretches the connective tissue."

That's the thing about therapeutic massage. It's not about legs and arms, butts, breasts and bellies. It's about muscles and bones and connective tissue and lymph. It's about coaxing the body into better alignment by relaxing the muscles that, in being held rigid, distort us—and releasing the repressions that distort us as well.

"So," I began, as he lifted my arm and began to massage my hand, "there are a couple of therapies I thought people might like to know about, such as hair analysis and food allergy testing."

"Hair analysis is something I have been using for about fifteen years. It was brought to my attention by an Arizona man under the care of Dr. Paul Eck. This man was in a mental institution. Dr. Eck tested his hair and administered vitamins and minerals. When I met the man he was totally recovered—selling vitamins, as a matter of fact.

"You send a sample of hair, and it is run through an atomic spectrophotometer. It's a mineral assay, such as used to determine minerals in drinking water. They check for very common minerals, like calcium, manganese, iron, magnesium, zinc, potassium and chromium. They also check for toxic metals like lead, or aluminum or arsenic."

The audio tape recorded a little yelp, as Gary dug into the muscle connecting my right shoulder to my neck.

"There are certain relationships between minerals, like potassium-calcium-magnesium that show up in a ratio. If the relationships are out of kilter, we give nutritional supplements to correct the imbalance.

"There was a boy, for instance, about eleven years old, whose mother brought him in because he was uncontrollable, always in fights, and said he was going to kill himself. We did a hair analysis, and gave him a few supplements he needed. He went on to be a football star and get his degree at the University of New Mexico. His mother says we literally saved his life."

"Mmmm." I was losing the ability to make cognitive comments as Gary's hands moved over my face, probing spots near my eyebrows and sliding down to my ears.

"Nowadays," he continued smoothly, gently pulling on my ears, "there are so many people who are aware of hair analysis. There is a medical doctor, a psychiatrist, who refers people to me to have their hair tested. These people have been in the psychiatric hospital. They all have pretty much the same kind of deficiency and need a certain kind of supplement."

I rallied slightly at the thought. "That implies mental illness has a physiological cause," I mumbled.

"It sure does. I could quote you many cases from my files where the right supplements brought people back to normal."

"In my particular case," I added more clearly, "a blood test showed acceptable calcium level, but the hair analysis recorded a deficiency. I suspect I was pulling calcium out of my bones and into the blood. Is that possible?"

"Sure. The other thing is, when you have a blood test, it shows the mineral levels in the blood at that particular moment. Hair analysis shows what is being absorbed by the cells over a longer period of time. It's like a statistical average. What is in the blood can fluctuate from daytime to nighttime, or from week to week, depending on other factors such as hormone levels."

How surprising that there could be such rapid fluctuations! The more I learn about the human body the more mystified I am at its complexity of interaction.

As Gary's hands continued to relax this body of mine, I wondered if they were sending chemical/electrical messages to all my precious little cells. My mental faculties were relaxing right along with the muscles. I was gradually being reduced to single sentences.

"Is there a relationship between the immune system and food allergies?"

"The immune system works on getting rid of materials in the blood that are damaged, imperfect or not functioning. It gets rid of debris, like dead cells and residues.

"One of the causes of food sensitivity is residue in the blood that the body can't use. A lot of times it has to do with poor assimilation, not enough digestive juices to thoroughly digest something. It may be an amino acid group that is small enough to pass through the intestinal walls, but too large for the cells of our body to assimilate and utilize in making proteins. When you have molecules that are too large, it's up to the immune system, the macrophages or the lymph cells, to digest or eliminate them.

"Most of the time people will develop sensitivity to food they are continually exposed to, food that they eat every day. If it's a processed food, or it's been cooked a long time, sometimes there is a deficiency of certain minerals or vitamins that the body needs to make enzymes required to digest those foods.

"So if there is a lack of those enzymes, the person doesn't thoroughly assimilate food and a residue builds up. It doesn't have to be food that is fatty or sugary. It might be a vegetable like a cucumber; maybe it's a tomato, maybe an onion. People might overeat a certain kind of food because they eat it constantly. When that happens, it does put stress on the immune system."

"How do you find out what food people are allergic to?"

"The most basic approach is a food elimination diet, where people keep a record of what they are eating. If they suspect something is causing trouble, they don't eat it for a couple of weeks. Then between meals, they eat some of it and record their reactions. If they get gas on their stomach or feel lousy, feel pain or need to go lie down, it's likely they are sensitive to that food.

"Another thing that I use is my little allertester, my little continuity tester."

"The same thing you use to measure the electrical resistance of the meridians?"

"Yes, that's what it is. The machine has an electromagnetic force field. You can put something on it, like an extract of food or solution containing pollen. If you put it on the tray and touch one of the reflex points, the meter can show if that allergen causes a problem. It really is very accurate."

I flopped over onto my stomach while Gary got some more massage oil. "Do your patients then eliminate the food or use a homeopathic remedy?"

"Both," he answered, rubbing the sweet smelling oil on my feet. "It's good to rotate foods, like every fourth day. And it's always good to have a variety, not to eat the same thing all the time."

"My children had scratch tests on their backs, but I have heard there's a blood test for allergies."

"There are actually two kinds of blood tests. With one, they just do a titre against immunoglobulin B. If that immunoglobulin is elevated there is hypersensitivity.

"The other kind of test is very expensive. They take a sample of blood and put a very minute drop of the blood on a slide. Next to it they place a drop of a suspected allergen, and then they just watch the blood under the microscope. They see if the blood goes away from that allergen, or goes with it."

"No kidding?" The idea raised my brain from lethargy. "As in 'Do I like you or do I not like you?'"

"Right! If it goes towards the substance it's OK. But if it runs away from it, that shows a violent reaction. It's as if the blood is saying, 'Go away from me, I don't want you!' They test for maybe 300 different things."

"Do you feel these blood tests are necessary, or can you do as well with your continuity tester?"

"I use my little tester because it's much faster, and I'm just looking for major allergies. Sometimes I have to go through all the little test vials to find out what are a patient's main allergies. If the meter shows a strong reaction, that's what we work on."

Gary went over to a shelf and got a special liniment to apply to my sore driving leg. I had just driven 1000 miles in two days, which I had not mentioned to him. He must have seen the energy blockage there.

"What do you think happens on a cellular level to cause cancer?" I asked, as he applied it to the back of my calf muscle. "Mmm, that smells different."

"My understanding is that when cells divide, the DNA molecule has to be reproduced. All the information of the whole body is in the DNA. Certain cells in the body do specific things. They are called differentiated cells. When cells divide, they are supposed to become the same kind of cells they were before. When there is something toxic in the body the cell can mutate. Actually what happens is the cell becomes undifferentiated, and doesn't know what to do."

I remembered Dr. Saiki telling me the cells forgot how to do their job and die, continually reproducing instead. But why, or how, does that happen? As Dr. Wong said, "If I knew that I would get the Nobel Prize!"

"Does it have something to do with the electrons?" I was prompting him to repeat something I'd half-forgotten from an earlier conversation.

"It might," he nodded, "because something that could cause the cell to mutate might be absorbing toxins that it cannot expel. Free radical ions, positively charged, combine with negatively charged electrons on the outside of the cell wall and take them away. This makes the cell lose its osmotic potential. It loses the ability to absorb nutrients and expel toxins."

"What are free radicals?"

"They are atoms or molecules which carry an unpaired electron and are highly reactive. They can come from many sources such as toxic chemicals, or rancid fats, or impure food. They can be inactivated by anti-oxidants, uric acid or certain enzymes.

"The immune system will recognize cells that are undifferentiated and will usually clean them up. The immune system is really intelligent. It can recognize cells that don't belong there. If we didn't have our immune systems our bodies would fill up with toxins in a matter of months.

"There is an article recently published in a science magazine that showed one of the things that causes weakness of the immune system is chlorinated water. Chlorine is good because it kills bacteria, but what are bacteria?"

I was about to mutter some sort of answer, but Gary went right ahead before I could get it out.

"Bacteria are single cell organisms, and chlorine kills single cell organisms. But what is our body made up of?"

I didn't even try to reply this time.

"...Trillions of cells. So if we have chlorine in our body and it kills some of these cells—and the immune system has the job of removing those cells—and we constantly drink chlorinated water, that stresses our immune system, weakening it."

"Do you believe the increase of toxins all around us, in food, air and water, account for the increase in cancer?" Gary was working on my back now. Massage on the back now felt great, ever since the time he pulled loose those adhesions.

"Yes. We have pollution in the air and water. Pollution in food comes from the various chemicals used in processing. They are not natural, they are synthetic, and our body just can't handle too much of them."

"Do you think a virus or bacteria starts the process of weakening the immune system?" My muffled voice sounded funny emanating from the donut shaped apparatus designed to keep my neck straight while he worked on my back.

"Sure. Any bacteria or virus that produces toxins can have an adverse effect on the function of our DNA. Cells will start mutating. If our immune system isn't strong enough to dispose of mutant cells, they will form a mass, a tumor."

"So how do we make our immune system function well enough to take care of them?" I pursued, raising my head for a breather.

"We have to be careful of the food we eat and the water we drink and thoughts we think—because the immune system understands language. If a person talks to himself and says, 'I want to be strong' or 'I feel good today,' that helps the immune system.

"If a person says 'Oh well, I don't feel good,' or 'I wish I were sick,'or 'I hurt,' then the immune system hears it and says 'Well, I guess we don't want to do much today. The boss says he doesn't want to feel good, so let's goof off.' "

It's the way affirmations work, that busy little voice in my head confirmed.

"That relates to another thing about going to see a doctor. If the doctor tells a patient he is sick and going to die in a year, it's really not good, because the doctor is a person of authority. What the doctor ought to say is 'Look, you should change your environment, you should change your habits; and if you don't change, but proceed the way you are right now, then you'll die in a year.' They don't think like that. A lot of doctors just look at the tests and tell patients they are going to die."

"They treat people the way they have been taught in medical school," I explained. "They use the standard procedures, like chemotherapy, but the best doctors add a dose of intuition and artful communication. I know from experience the power of authority is tremendous. We believe what doctors tell us as if it were absolute truth. Maybe our immune systems believe it too, and every cell in our body hears that pronouncement." Considering my state of relaxation, that was quite a speech for me.

Gary picked up on my mention of chemotherapy. "Chemotherapy

treats the body like cancer is an invasion. So we are going to kill cancer cells. But the chemotherapy cripples our immune system."

"That's the question I asked Dr. McIver, when he told me I would need to have chemotherapy. 'Why not enhance the immune system, instead?'"

"What did he answer?"

"He said perhaps some day that will be possible, but now the best treatment available is chemotherapy, and the immune system always recovers."

"Well, our immune systems are indeed remarkable. They can kill cancer cells; they can do it on their own. That's why some people can have spontaneous remissions. It really can happen.

"For instance they can go to a faith healer, someone they really believe in, really strongly believe in. If that person says, 'You are truly healed,' then sometimes they actually are cured. It's because the immune system will respond to that."

"The immune system must also respond to subconscious thoughts we are not even aware of," I volunteered. Thank you, Dottee, Diane, Alton, for helping me understand that concept too.

"Absolutely. My personal idea is that there is a spirit in the world that wants us to succeed, that wants us to be happy. I call it God. Some people alienate from that spirit, doing things that are self-destructive.

"If we tune in to that spirit, it makes us feel whole. That's what some people call grace, or faith. It's what makes us feel complete.

"Emotional environment has a lot to do with our state of being. If people are happy, complete, in a situation where they don't experience stress; and they feel purposeful, doing something valuable, it actually helps their immune systems. It augments the energy needed to heal themselves."

"So it's a good idea to have a purpose, to have fun and enjoy yourself. I always suspected it was, but felt guilty about doing it."

"It is good."

"A lot of the very negative things we are taught to believe about ourselves very early in life, when we don't realize what we are learning, work to the detriment of our bodies, immune systems and spirits," I suggested, feeling mentally inspired by Gary's hands massaging my back.

"That's right. Much of what we are talking about has to do with thought. Everything we are, really, is what we have thought about. **Many** times people are hypnotized into accepting something that is not true. That's why it is important to meditate, so that we can actually become de-hypnotized—so we are not being controlled and manipulated."

"How does that work?"

"Meditation helps people get an overview of their whole life, to gain perspective of themselves and everyone around them. It's actually what I consider a kind of atonement—at-one-ment with everything. Tuning in.

"When people are really tuned in to the world, someone could knock on the door and they would know who it is before they open it. Someone would call on the telephone and they would know who was calling before they picked up the receiver. And when they were talking to that person on the phone, they would intuitively know where that person was calling from, even what kind of clothes that person was wearing. It's as if they are so in tune with everything around them they can pick up on these things."

"I think," I said, lifting my face for air again, "that we all have glimmerings of that from time to time. Some people seem to be able to do it consistently."

"Some people think it is beyond our human capability to have that kind of awareness. But to me, that's what experiencing reality is all about. When you know what's real, and you know what is appropriate to do at that time, then you're in tune."

I felt pretty well tuned in to Gary's thought processes at that moment. "If you are in that state, it must be what people call a state of grace."

"That's it," he proceeded enthusiastically, "that's the state of enlightenment! Down through the ages, people who were considered to be Masters had that energy, that spirit, in which they are able to be aware of everything. Tuned in."

I may not have reached enlightenment, but I was indeed feeling warm, expansive, energized. "What we're tuning in to is, in addition to our seen world, an unseen world that has an effect on us because it must be a part of us."

"Yes. But there's a lot more. There are forces like magnetism. We live in a world that is held in space by a magnetic force field that we don't see or feel. But we experience it, for it keeps us on the planet, and keeps our planet rotating around the sun at a certain speed. Our planet has kept rotating at a certain speed for millions of years, all because of forces we can't see. That's awesome, when you think about it!

"Why not work with these forces within our body? Why not be aware of them? Because they do exist."

Gary patted my shoulder to signal he was finished with the massage, spent a moment with closed eyes balancing my aura, then quietly left the room.

I lay there in complete relaxation for a few moments, as my thoughts wandered on. Why not, indeed? That's what healing techniques are all about. Massage, shamanic counseling, nutrition, homeopathy, sound, acupuncture—even surgery, oncology, radiation—they are all working with these forces that we don't see, but which do exist.

Reaching lazily for my clothes, I resolved to continue my course of learning, my transformational journey. Not that I could really stop it! I knew those unseen forces would see to it that I kept moving forward, by pushing, pulling, beckoning, enticing, shoving, tripping, supporting and embracing me on that unpaved path.

"Guess we're committed, Cynthia," my friend Intellect whispered in my ear. "Better get up and get at it!"

"OK, OK," I answered her, under my breath, "I'm coming…one foot after the other…one moment at a time. But please don't push!" So I paid my bill, hugged Gary (who was used to it by that time) and left Adventureland, ready for the next part of my journey, whatever it might prove to be.

Traveling Companions

Who knows where the road will take me now? I've traveled a long way on this journey back to wellness. But where have I arrived?

My doctors say I am in "remission." According to *The Random House Dictionary of the English Language* it means "a temporary or permanent decrease or subsidence of manifestations of a disease." "Remission" is a cautious term; usually understood to imply that there will be, at some point in time, a recurrence of disease.

There is another way to describe the place I am in: the awesome word, "cure." According to the same source, cure is "successful remedial treatment; restoration to health."

I consider myself cured!

Why? Because I am far more than suppressed symptoms—I have sought out and exposed their cause to light. My body has received the best treatment Western medicine has to offer, and through alternative therapies my mind and spirit have been restored to balance. That fulfills, on an emotional and physical level, Random House's definition of health.

I imagine that I am, symbolically, a biathlon athlete, rowing on the River of Belief, towards the shore where I mount my Bicycle of Earnest Endeavor, cycling down the Road to Enlightenment, passing through the City of Hope into the State of Wholeness.

It's the best kind of biathlon—no competition, except from occasional sputtering Fears, Uncertainties and Doubts that pop up from time to time, testing resolve.

"That's OK," Intellect tells me. "Don't fret about those FUDs. It's part of being human. You're still moving forward. I'm with you every step of the way."

And oh, what an Olympic cheering section supports me on my way! Many people have handed me symbolic cups of water and snacks, or practical advice and information. They have been with me from the start, companions on my journey.

Those healers whom you have already met are major cheerleaders, but also rooting me on are just good friends like Mary, Betty, Teresa, Grace, Celesta, and Karol.

Behind the scenes, the Layerist network and prayer groups like Mother's church and Silent Unity work on an unseen level. And perhaps most important, a river of healing love and support flows continually from my husband, my mother, my children and all the other members of our extended families.

But not everyone is as blessed as I. What if you feel you are alone? In that case, you need to realize that everyone has someone, even if they don't know it. We are all connected, in a way far beyond our understanding.

Reach out! Bring in that healing love! Make the initial effort to connect! Call your doctor, local hospitals and the American Cancer Society to locate support groups! Walk into the nearest church or synagogue or mosque or ashram, even if you don't belong, and ask for healing prayers!

Read Bernie Siegel and Deepak Chopra and Louise Hayes and more of the many helpful authors whose works are listed in the resource section of this book. Listen to their tapes. Open your mind. They will be your cheerleaders.

Believe in your body's ability to heal! If you feel your body has betrayed you, do what you can to fix it, and practice radical trust. Affirm! Affirm hope and healing!

A car that develops a broken water pump doesn't get discarded in a junk yard—it gets fixed and put back on the road for many more good years of service. You may have to clean out the radiator and fuel lines and replace a few worn parts, but in the end it becomes a serviceable vehicle again.

Above all, do not cringe in paralyzing fear. Fear of pain, fear of death, fear of hurting others, causing others pain, fear of loss, fear of failure—the list goes on forever. Fears are very powerful, but they are nothing except negative fantasizing. Neutralize them with trust. Radical trust!

Grow and learn and increase your awareness until the point, which comes to all of us at some time, when we actually do undertake that death journey into life. Then we will no longer have separation to bar us from reunion with our Source, bliss and inestimable joy.

This is not to say our road is without potholes. Those are the times when we call upon our invisible travelling companions, who are always available to help us. I know about them now, in a way I did not before.

You might call them imagination, but I call them makers of miracles. Every time I have hit the depths of despair during this past five years, (and quite often I was in those valleys) I surrendered, asked, and minor miracles brought me solace.

Like the time during chemotherapy I begged the Virgin Mary for help—and felt an unmistakable blazing energy flow from toes to head.

And like when we found the arrowheads. Ted and I have walked hundreds of miles out on our mesa, scrutinizing the ground for artifacts. There isn't much to find, because people have been hunting arrowheads, just as we do, for centuries. In ten years of searching, we have only found two or three.

But one night, when I was particularly despondent, I prayed for a sign that someone was looking after me. The next day Ted and I walked into an area we had not visited before. Right on top of a sandy hollow by a piñon tree, as fresh as if it were placed there yesterday, was a perfectly formed black arrowhead. Wow! What a gift! It joined Na-tan, the bear, by my bedside.

You can say it was coincidence, and I thought a little about that too. So we got further confirmation. The very next day Ted and I went looking again. This time Ted found a perfectly formed, translucent white arrowhead. It joined the black one by my bear.

Thanks guys, I believe! Two days in a row, black and white, yin and yang, alpha and omega—it bends the boundaries of coincidence.

Another day, encouraged by this reinforcement (Oh! how the spirits must shake their heads at the brazenness of this soul) I walked the mesa alone with our dogs, wrestling with the decision of whether to build our house in Colorado. There were a lot of good fear-based reasons not to. It would eat up all our savings; maybe I would get sick again; perhaps we were too old to deal with mud and snow and bad roads; maybe mother would suffer from such major change; suppose we weren't up to starting all over; how could we bring in electricity, get hooked up to a water supply, build from scratch.

Counterbalancing the fear was my life-long dream. Beautiful vistas, crystal clean air, tall pines, birds, elk, deer, bear, sunrises, sunsets, stars, peacefulness, harmony, ecstasy of nature.

"All right, Great Grand Director," I pleaded, "I need another sign. If it is the right path for us to take, please show me a red arrowhead!"

(Is there no end to my impertinence?)

Not only do you almost never find arrowheads, you especially almost never find *red* arrowheads. I knew I was asking a lot, but I walked along chirpily chanting "Red arrowhead, red arrowhead—if I should go ahead, show me red arrowhead."

You guessed it. Right by a dried snakeweed bush lay a red arrowhead. It was not perfect. It was broken, but it was definitely a red arrowhead. Next day I signed the papers and wiped out my bank account. Last summer, we started building our new home, and somehow everything we need appears.

Another small miracle of confirmation about the house occurred when the bear pooped on my altar up there in the woods. (At least I chose to see it as confirmation.)

Remember the story of the sun spinning at Fatima? Thousands of people saw it. One evening just before sundown, I was walking in our Colorado woods while Ted was cooking supper on the camping grill. I noticed that the shafts of sunlight slanting through the pines seemed different; so I walked to a clearing by the road, looking to the west. Around the setting sun, many-colored radiating circles of light shimmered and spun.

"Ted, come here!" I hollered. He came running, probably thinking I had encountered the resident bear. "Do you see it too?" I was wondering if it were my eyesight, or my imagination, or if it just possibly might be true.

Ted observed a few moments, quietly confirmed it, shook his head in wonder. Curiously enough, Betty Rice had been out walking 500 miles away in Arizona the same afternoon. She told me the sun was spinning there too.

And then there was the time when I was really down once again, and the face of Jesus appeared in my marbleized washbasin. No kidding.

You know that black and white picture with splotches all over it that seems like nothing—until you change your focus, and there is the face of Jesus gazing at you? Well this was the same kind of thing. I wondered why I had never seen it before. A couple days later it was gone, and I never have been able to find it again, no matter how hard I try.

So what is going on? Either I get the Nobel Prize for imagination, or something really is happening on unseen levels. Somewhat to my relief, it is going on in the lives of others as well.

As an example, Teresa telephoned one morning, in awe that her grandmother's silver rosary had turned to gold overnight, during a meditative mountain retreat. The same has been occurring to rosaries among pilgrims to Medjugorge. It is a real phenomenon, which nobody has been able to explain.

These are only a few of the many minor miracles that have occurred. They seem to be increasing as time goes on. There really is something out there that wants to help and guide us. Maybe they are angels. Whatever you want to call them, they are our invisible traveling companions.

They guide us by means of dreams, as well. Listen to them. Whenever you have an especially vivid dream, write it down immediately and consult a good dream analysis book like Wilda Tanner's *The Mystical, Magical, Marvelous World of Dreams.* Look up the symbols. They are signposts to the messages from your unconscious allies, or your unconscious self.

The nature of our life journey is that we move forward; but sometimes we are not aware of our progress. The only way we can see how far we have come is to look back at where we have been.

I am looking back now.

Five years ago, I was an entirely different person, on every level. Not a single atom that was in my body then is there today. I believe it.

When Ted shakes his head and says "Cynthia, you are a difficult woman!" I give him a hug and smile with pleasure, because it means I have left the compliant, please-everybody, "nice" person I was behind. I am still a loving, caring person; but I love and care about myself too, these days.

Five years ago I was embarrassed to say to Ted that I was going to meditate. That was too spooky a word at the time. I told him I was going to lie down for a rest instead.

Five years ago I felt we should be in agreement in everything we did. This was just being a good wife. Now I know his agenda and mine are often different, and I don't feel I have to be part of his every activity; nor he, a part of mine.

In the past four and a half years I have neutralized a lot of anger, hurt and resentment, through awareness sparked by my healers. I have brought up the feelings, understood the lessons they were teaching me, and learned to practice forgiveness—of myself as well as others.

Five years ago I would never have seen an acupuncturist, a naturopath, a nutritionist, a color therapist, or—worse even—a shaman.

Now I have a standing weekly acupuncture appointment. I check in regularly for massage. And without a shred of guilt I participate in other alternative healing processes, from craniosacral therapy to the ancient, sacred mysteries of the Native American sweat lodge.

Since the time Celesta read me out on the astral level and talked me into making a five year plan, I have committed to building our home in the wilderness, bought a computer and written this book. I have learned to ski, to do Reiki and practice Tai Chi Chih. I have traveled to renew friendships from my youth, from California to Nova Scotia, attended workshops, visited my children and grandchildren, had lots of fun. It has all been part of my journey back to wellness.

Who says serious illness is the end of living? It is just the beginning! It makes you realize that life is not to be wasted. Life is to be enjoyed, with zest and delight! It is an oh-so-precious invitation to growth and learning.

The opportunity to make this journey into living is going to exist for an awful lot of women. Over two years ago, when I started writing this book, breast cancer struck one woman in nine. Currently, the statistics have been revised to one in eight. And men are getting it too.

Maybe soon medical research will find a physical cure. But until then, there is hope, and there are always choices for courses of action. For one thing, we can decide how we want to perceive our illness and the world—the time-worn "pitcher is half empty or half full" routine.

There are other curative methods available to us now. Healing is not just remission. It is clearing out the garbage of mind, body and spirit, and bringing those elements into balance and harmony. There are many new as well as ancient ways to do that, and that's where alternative therapies come in, working with modern medical wizardry for cure. Restoration to health.

However, in the end, who is the real healer? Until I was ready, until someone held a mirror up to me, I still didn't quite get it.

Sometimes the most astonishing insights come from "chance" encounters, if there really is such a thing as a chance encounter. I was in Toronto, celebrating my sixty-first birthday by visiting my son Michael, who was appearing as one of Donny Osmond's brothers in "Joseph and the Amazing Technicolor Dream Coat."

The show was at the beautifully restored Elgin Theatre. At intermission, a young woman came to my seat and introduced herself as Lori MacLean, a friend of Michael's. She was manager of the "house," overseeing the ushers and making sure everything was running smoothly.

Would I like to see something special during intermission? Of course. So she took me upstairs, into a whole different theatre, the Winter Garden, directly above the Elgin, that had been walled off and forgotten for decades.

Such a place of enchantment! Still decorated for the last performance of "A Midsummer Night's Dream," the ceiling was hung with leafy branches and twinkling lanterns. Pastoral scenes decorated the stage canopy and walls. Columns had been transformed into gnarled tree trunks. It felt like being in a leafy bower. Was Puck hiding behind one of those trees, ready to play his tricks?

We stood at the orchestra rail, delighting in the magic of the place, conversing in hushed tones. Two strangers, instantly bonded, plunging into intense exchange.

I told her about my breast cancer and the book I was writing. Her enthusiasm for my project lifted me higher.

"How many healers are you going to write about?" Lori asked.

"Eight." I named each of them.

"There ought to be nine," she stated emphatically. "You should include yourself as a healer."

"Why me?" I spluttered, astonished at the idea.

"Think about it," came her cryptic reply.

I did. It only took a minute for the light to dawn.

Yes, Lori was absolutely right. Others can help you, show you the way, open your mind, change your body; but in the final analysis—on the deepest, most profound level—you heal yourself.

So I guess I have become a healer after all!

List of Resources

These books and tapes were helpful to me personally as I moved along the path to recovery. There is much more of value out there. Any inquiry will lead to a wealth of information and discovery. So inquire! If a book listed is no longer in print at the time you read this, try locating it through your public library. They are often able to find it locally, or through their inter-library loan systems.

A C U P U N C T U R E

In the United States, regulation of acupuncture and Oriental medicine differs from state to state. To determine the status of acupuncture in your state, or to locate a licensed acupuncturist near you, contact either your state's Licensing Board through the Department of Health, or:

> The National Certification Commission for Acupuncturists
> 1424 16th Street, Suite 501
> Washington, D.C. 20036
> (202) 232-1404

Manaka, Yoshio, M.D. & Urquhart, Ian A., Ph.D.; *The Layman's Guide To Acupuncture;* John Weatherhill, Inc., 149 Madison Ave., New York, NY 10016

Mann, Felix, M.B.; *Acupuncture,* Revised Edition; Random House, Inc.; 201 East 50th St., New York, NY 10022

B O D Y W O R K

For information about massage therapy, or to locate a licensed massage therapist in your area, contact

> The American Massage Therapy Association
> 820 Davis Street, Suite 100
> Evanston, IL 60201-4444
> (708) 864-0123

John Feltman, Editor; *Hands-On Healing—Massage Remedies For Hundreds Of Health Problems;* Rodale Press; 33 East Minor St., Emmaus, PA 18098

AMERICAN CANCER SOCIETY. call 1-800-227-2345 to find local office. Your local office can provide information on available programs, area support groups; literature on chemotherapy, radiation, etc.

NATIONAL CANCER INSTITUTE. For information and referral service, or information on current clinical trials, call 1-800-4-CANCER.

Anderson, Greg; *The Cancer Conqueror*; Andrews and McMeel; 4900 Main Street, Kansas City, MO 64112

Buchanan, Sue; *Surviving Breast Cancer—Love, Laughter and a High Disregard for Statistics*; Thomas Nelson Publishers; P.O. Box 141000, Nashville, Tennessee 37214; 1-800-251-4000

Love, Susan M.; *Dr. Susan Love's Breast Book*; Addison-Wesley Publishing Co., Inc.; Route 128, Redding, MA 01867; 1-800-447-2226

Lynes, Barry; *The Cancer Cure that Worked*; published in Canada by Marcus Books, P.O. Box 327, Queensville, Ont., Canada L0G IR0, (416) 478-2201; FAX (416) 478-8338

—*The Healing of Cancer*; Marcus Books, address above

—*Helping the Cancer Victim*; Marcus Books, address above

NOTE: To order any of Barry Lynes books listed above, call 1-800-245-5445 (Summit University Press)

Moss, Ralph W., Ph.D.; *Cancer Therapy—The Independent Consumer's Guide To Non-toxic Treatment And Prevention*; Equinox Press; 331 West 57th Street, Suite 268, New York, NY 10019; (212) 245-4639

Siegel, Bernie S., M.D.; *Love, Medicine And Miracles*; Harper and Row Publishers, Inc.; 10 East 53rd Street, New York, NY 10022

C O L O R & G E M S T O N E S

Mella, Dorothee L.; *Stone Power*; Warner Books; 666 Fifth Avenue, New York, NY 10103, or Domel Publications; P.O. Box 3829, Albuquerque, NM 87110

—The Language of Color; Warner Books or Domel Publications, addresses above

—Candle Power, "Tote-a-Book"; Domel Publications, address above

—Color Your Meals Nutritious; Domel Publications, address above

—Functional Color A to Z, "Tote-a-Book"; Domel Publications, address above

—Gem Pharmacy, "Tote-a-Book"; Domel Publications, address above

—Colors for Healing; Domel Publications, address above

C O N S C I O U S N E S S

Monroe, Robert; *Journeys out of the Body;* Doubleday; 1540 Broadway, New York, NY 10036; 1-800-223-6834

—Far Journeys; Doubleday; address above

—Ultimate Journey; Doubleday; address above

—The Monroe Institute; Route 1, Box 175; Faber, VA 22938-9749

D R E A M S

Crisp, Tony; *Dream Dictionary;* Wings Books, distributed by Outlet Book Company, 40 Engelhard Ave., Avenel, NJ 07001

Tanner, Wilda B.; *The Mystical, Magical, Marvelous World of Dreams;* Sparrow Hawk Press, P.O. Box 1274, Tahlequah, OK 74465

H E R B S

Tierra, Michael, C.A., N.D.; *The Way of Herbs;* Pocket Books, A division of Simon and Schuster; 1230 Avenue of the Americas, New York, NY 10020

Weiner, Michael A., Ph.D. and Janet A.; *Herbs that Heal;* Quantum Books; 6 Knoll Lane, Mill Valley, CA 94941

Brennan, Barbara Ann; *Hands of Light—A Guide to Healing through the Human Energy Field;* Bantam Books; 666 Fifth Avenue, New York, NY 10103

Chopra, Deepak, M.D.; *Quantum Healing;* Bantam Books; 1540 Broadway, New York, NY 10036

—*Perfect Health—The Complete Mind/Body Guide;* Harmony Books; 201 East 50th St., New York, NY 10022

Cousins, Norman; *Head First—The Biology of Hope and the Healing Power of the Human Spirit;* Penguin Books U.S.A.; 375 Hudson Street, New York, NY 10014

—*Anatomy of an Illness;* Bantam Books, published by arrangement with W.W. Norton & Co., Inc.; 500 Fifth Avenue, New York, NY 10110

Gawain, Shakti; *Creative Visualization;* New World Library; 58 Paul Drive, San Rafael, CA 94903

—*Living in the Light;* New World Library; address above

Hay, Louise L.; *You Can Heal Your Life;* Hay House, Inc.; 1154 E. Dominguez Street, P.O. Box 6204, Carson, CA 90749-6204

—*The Power Is within You;* Hay House, address above

King, Serge; *Imagineering for Health—Self-Healing through the Use of the Mind;* a Quest book; The Theosophical Publishing House; 306 West Geneva Road, Wheaton, IL 60187

—*Kahuna Healing;* The Theosophical Publishing House; address above

Kubler-Ross, Elisabeth; *On Death and Dying;* Collier Books, Macmillan Publishing Co.; 866 Third Avenue, New York, NY 10022

Lieberman, Jacob, O.D., Ph.D.; *Light, Medicine of the Future;* Bear and Co.; Santa Fe, NM 87504-2860

Locke, Steven, M.D., and Colligan, Douglas; *The Healer Within—the New Medicine of Mind and Body;* E.P. Dutton, a division of New American Library; 2 Park Avenue, New York, NY 10016

MEDITATION

Young, Shinzen, *Five Classic Meditations,* (audio tape); Audio Renaissance Tapes, Inc.; 5858 Wilshire Boulevard, Suite 205, Los Angeles, CA 90036; 1-800-221-7945

MUSIC

Focal Point; *Inner Peace Meditation;* (audio tape); Genesis Reflection; P.O. Box 4111, Simi Valley, CA 93093

—*Alpha Meditation,* (audio tape); Genesis Reflection; address above

NATUROPATHY

For information and the location of medical doctors who specialize in natural therapies near you, contact:

American Naturopathic Medical Association
P.O. Box 96273, Las Vegas, NV 89193
(702) 897-7053

Turner, Roger Newman, N.D., B.Ac., M.B.N.O.A.; *Naturopathic Medicine—Treating the Whole Person;* Thorsons Publishers, Ltd.; Wellingsborough, Northamptonshire, England

NUTRITION

To obtain information about orthomolecular medicine or to locate a specialist in clinical nutrition in your area, contact

The Canadian Schizophrenia Foundation *(also known as the International Society for Orthomolecular Medicine)*
16 Florence Avenue,
Toronto, Ontario, Canada M2N 1E9
(416) 733-2117

Diamond, Harvey and Marilyn; *Fit for Life;* Warner Books; 666 5th Avenue, New York, NY 10103

Hausman, Patricia, and Hurley, Judith Benn; *The Healing Foods—the Ultimate Authority on the Creative Power of Nutrition;* Dell Publishing; 666 Fifth Avenue, New York, NY 10103

Morningstar, Amadea, with Urmilla Desai; *The Ayurvedic Cookbook, A Personalized Guide to Good Nutrition and Health;* Lotus Press; P.O. Box 6265, Santa Fe, NM 87502

Robbins, John; *Diet for a New America;* Stillpoint Publishing; Box 640, Walpole, NH 03608; 1-800-847-4014

P R A Y E R

Contact any church, synagogue, mosque, ashram, etc., as they have prayer groups which can remember you in their prayers

Silent Unity; Unity Village, MO 64065; (816) 246-5400, 24 hours a day

S E L F   I M P R O V E M E N T

Borysenko, Joan, Ph.D.; *Guilt is the Teacher, Love is the Lesson;* Warner Books; 1271 Avenue of the Americas, New York, NY 10020

—*Minding the Body, Mending the Mind;* Warner Books, address above

Bradshaw, John; *Healing the Shame that Binds You;* Health Communications, Inc.; Enterprise Venter, 3201 SW 15th St., Deerfield Beach, FL 33442

Jampolsky, Gerald G., M.D.; *Love Is Letting Go of Fear;* Celestial Arts; P.O. Box 7327, Berkeley, CA 94707

—*Feel the Fear and Do it Anyway;* Celestial Arts, address above

John-Roger and McWilliams, Peter; *You Can't Afford the Luxury of a Negative Thought;* Prelude Press; 8159 Santa Monica Boulevard, Los Angeles, CA 90046; 1-800-LIFE-101

Kabat-Zinn, Jon, Ph.D.; *Full Catastrophe Living;* Delacorte Press, Bantam Doubleday Dell Publishing Group, Inc.; 666 Fifth Avenue, New York, NY 10103

Williamson, Marianne; *A Woman's Worth;* Random House; New York, NY 10022; paperback edition, Ballentine Books, New York, NY

Achterburg, Joan; *Imagery in Healing—Shamanism and Modern Medicine*; Shambala Publications, Inc.; Horticultural Hall, 300 Massachusetts Avenue, Boston, MA 02115

Halifax, Joan; *Shamanic Voices; a Survey of Visionary Narratives*; Viking Penguin; 375 Hudson Street, New York, NY 10014; 1-800-331-4624

Harner, Michael; *The Way of the Shaman*; Harper San Francisco, a division of Harper Collins Publishers; 10 East 53rd Street, New York, NY 10022

Ingerman, Sandra; *Soul Retrieval—Mending the Fragmented Self*; Harper San Francisco; address above

King, Serge; *Mastering Your Hidden Self—A Guide to the Huna Way*; A Quest Book; The Theosophical Publishing House; 306 West Geneva Road, Wheaton, IL 60187

Nicholson, Shirley; *Shamanism—An Expanded View of Reality*; A Quest book; The Theosophical Publishing House; 306 West Geneva Road, Wheaton, IL 60187

S U R G E R Y

Boyd, Gary; *Coping with Surgery: a Guide to Self Help*; Heritage Associates, Inc; P.O. Box 6291, Albuquerque, NM 87197

How to Survive Chemotherapy
for breast cancer with a maximum
of comfort and ease

Chemotherapy is not fun, but it is a valid way to fight cancer and there are many things I learned to do to make it easier. These helpful hints are things I discovered in my own therapy or were passed on to me from others.

Physical Side Effects of Chemotherapy

MOUTH SORES

I significantly reduced the frequency and severity of mouth sores with the following dental hygiene, starting as soon as I had my first chemotherapy:

—I brushed my teeth after every meal, using a soft toothbrush and an oxygenating dental powder such as Vince, or toothpaste such as Mentadent. They can be found in drug stores and most supermarkets.

—Before brushing, I used dental floss to clean out food particles from between the teeth. I was careful not to injure the gums in flossing.

—After brushing, I brushed again with pure aloe gel and swished it all around my mouth. I spit the excess, but did not rinse it out. The gel is tasteless and not unpleasant to use.

—I was careful to avoid injury to the mouth with harsh, scratchy foods. It's not that I couldn't eat them, I just ate them carefully, as the tissue lining the mouth was fragile from chemo.

—If sores did develop, I bought some large chewable vitamin C lozenges, 500 mg., and sucked one several times a day, letting the fluid bathe the affected area as long as possible. This often reduced the severity and duration of the sores.

THROAT PAIN

Avoiding throat pain was easier than curing it. After eating and before bedtime I sipped a tablespoon of food quality aloe liquid. I did not eat or drink for a while afterwards to allow the aloe to soothe the throat.

I used an over-the-counter hydrocortisone ointment such as Caldecort, inserting it gently after each bowel movement. When the irritation was severe, my doctor prescribed a cortisone suppository, which is stronger. I found the irritation was in the sphincter muscle, so in using the suppository I simply held it in place a few moments then removed it. That way the medication went where the problem was, not above it where it didn't do a lot of good.

I made sure my diet included plenty of fiber from fresh vegetables, fruits and grains.

N A U S E A

My doctor prescribed various anti-nausea medications, which were very helpful and good. I found that sipping ginger ale was helpful; also eating small amounts more frequently. There is a Jamaican-style ginger ale available at health food stores or nutrition centers which has less sugar and more spice than that which we normally drink. It is very effective in calming the stomach. I mixed it with papaya. The papaya juice is easy to digest. Saltine crackers were good for settling the stomach. I followed my intuition—what sounded good felt good in my stomach.

H A I R

People on aggressive chemotherapy will almost surely lose their hair. Mine began to fall out about two or two and a half weeks after my first chemotherapy. Most of it fell out at that time, but wisps remained, gradually falling out over the following months. It grew back after chemo ended, but in the meantime there wasn't much I could do except buy a wig and turbans or caps before it fell out. I realized I am much more than my appearance, even though all body hair disappeared.

I N F E C T I O N S

Because chemotherapy weakened my immune system by lowering my white blood cell count I was more susceptible than normal to infections. So I avoided crowds, stayed away from people with colds, and limited my contact with children, especially during the period halfway between chemo courses when my white count was lowest. When I ran a fever, I contacted my doctor immediately.

I practiced frequent hand-washing. I always washed my hands before eating food, and always when coming home after being out in public, handling groceries, etc. I washed my food, too, when practical. Who knew if the grocery clerk had sneezed when stacking up the tomatoes?

Good perineal care was important too, in order to avoid bladder infections. I used a squirt bottle with water in it to wash the vaginal area whenever I went to the bathroom.

DIARRHEA

When I developed diarrhea, my doctor prescribed medication to control it. But I handled mild cases myself by temporarily eating low-fiber foods high in complex carbohydrates, such as pasta, potatoes or rice. An old Polish remedy in my husband's family is to dissolve 2 heaping tablespoons of corn starch in a half cup tepid water and drink it. It does not taste bad, and is soothing and nourishing. I repeated it as often as I needed.

SKIN CARE

I used a natural, aloe-based body lotion after bathing in order to keep skin moist and comfortable. Aloe is such a good friend!

MUSCLE WEAKNESS & TENDERNESS

My muscles and tendons became weak and easily damaged. The best treatment I found was prevention. Exercise was helpful, but it had to be gentle, not stressful. Walking was my best exercise and had the added benefits of fresh air and sunshine. I was careful not to strain by lifting or carrying heavy objects, twisting or jerking. I got plenty of rest; napped when possible. Those muscles really appreciated the opportunity to heal. I stretched my arm on the side of surgery every day to avoid atrophy. A good time to do it was when it was warm from a bath or shower, reaching gently above my head and leaving the arm there for 30 seconds at a time. I was careful not to jerk, for that can tear the muscles, causing micro damage that is hard to heal.

S U P P O R T — S U P P O R T —
S U P P O R T — S U P P O R T —
S U P P O R T — S U P P O R T —
S U P P O R T —

There are many ways in which people can take an active part in their own healing and support the care given by doctors. I checked them out. I have written about some of them in this book, but there are many others. It is important to use good judgment and investigate them thoroughly, and combine them with allopathic treatment following your doctor's advice. Here are some of my thoughts about supportive therapies:

N U T R I T I O N

A good nutritionist helps to maintain the strength and body weight needed to stand up to chemotherapy. He or she analyzes the patient's medical history, takes blood samples and suggests a diet and regimen of vitamins and food supplements tailored to individual needs.

A C U P U N C T U R E

Because acupuncture works on an energy level, it can be very helpful in keeping energy up. It can also relieve stress and nausea and just make people feel better.

I N V O L V E M E N T

At some point, when people have become accustomed to the structure and effects of chemotherapy, it is important to set future goals that involve being here and actively participating in life. People benefit from acting on their plans to paint that picture or build that dream house or write that book or set up a network to help others in the same situation. Involvement and purpose create energy and a reason to hang around. It also makes cancer patients easier people to be with.

S U P P O R T   G R O U P S

Those who have a very supportive circle of friends are fortunate. There are various support groups for cancer patients, and also for spouses. These groups supply emotional support, as well as information and practical assistance. The local office of the American Cancer Society has information about them.

I found it was important to do things that gave me pleasure and avoid things and people that drained my energy. I could not allow any negativity around me. Negativity feeds fear and fear restricts healing. I surrounded myself with positive people and positive thoughts. I tried to develop my relationship with a higher power, which means different things to different people. I visualized my cancer cells being eaten by Pac-men or bugs or tigers. I visualized my healing light penetrating my body. I rested my body in sleep or meditation. I deliberately chose colors to wear that made me feel good (pinks are self-nurturing, greens are healing). I got out in nature as much as possible. I met with friends, watched funny movies, breathed deeply, hugged my pets and sang! Singing opens up channels for joy.

Helpful Hints for Radiation Therapy

The following were helpful to me while undergoing radiation:

I wore loose, soft, comfortable clothes that are easy to get in and out of. I did not wear a bra until treatment was finished.

I protected the irradiated area from sunlight by covering it up with clothing and wearing a hat.

I tried to maintain structure and order around myself. I avoided stress and got plenty of rest. I wore healing colors and carried banded gemstones to help preserve order in my electromagnetic field.

After each radiation treatment, I slathered pure aloe gel on the treated parts. I was told by the nurses not to use ordinary creams or lotions that might contain minerals or metals. I did not put anything on my skin before each treatment, but waited until afterwards.

I bathed nightly in comfortably warm (not hot) water, to which was added a pound of sea salt and a pound of baking soda. This soothes the skin and is supposed to pull out toxins. It's also good for the spirit.

I devised a healing metaphor for the radiation ray. In my case it was rays from the hands of Jesus, but it could be the aurora borealis, or the sun goddess or a laser beam like in Star Wars. I saw it destroying only cancer cells. I imagined that what it did not destroy, it illuminated and cleansed.

I nurtured myself. I surrounded myself with positivity and avoided negativity. I was the most important person in the world right then! I did whatever made me feel bliss, guilt-free!

Index

lentil and ginger soup, 197
leucocyte, 77
leukemia, 73, 81, 85, 201, 209
lifestyle, 30-31, 57, 79, 86, 100
lifetimes, other, 199
light, 6, 19, 38, 40, 45-47, 49, 57, 62, 78, 84, 95, 99, 123, 129-130, 132-136, 138, 140, 142-144, 146, 148, 150, 152, 154, 159, 167, 185, 187, 197, 219, 221-224, 226, 228, 230, 247, 250, 253, 258-259, 266
linear accelerator, 132, 134, 143

loss, 15, 48, 76, 80, 117, 121-123, 208, 248
love, 9, 15, 17-18, 25, 46-47, 50-51, 62, 66, 104, 113, 129, 162, 168, 171, 179, 188, 191, 195, 200, 227, 248, 251, 256, 260-261, motherly, 136, the child within, 67, 163, unconditional, 35
lower world, 190
lumpectomy, 22-23, 145
lymph glands, 13, 23, 133, 142, 145-146, 201
lymph nodes, 13, 18, 25, 55, 145-146
lymph system, 14
lymphatics, 145-149
lymphoma, 73, 142
Lynes, Barry, 219-220, 256

M

MRI, 141
malignant, 22, 75, 78, 87, 135, 157
mammogram, 13, 29, 31-32, 88, 185
mammography, 26, 87
Mana, 104
mandrake, 209-210
margins, 23, 145-146
marriage, 110, 175
Mary, Virgin, 249
massage, 7, 105-106, 119, 154, 159, 222-230, 235, 237-238, 240, 242, 246, 252, 255-256
mastectomy, modified radical, 16, 22-23, 133
mastectomy, radical, 21-24

mastectomy bra, 59
mastitis, 27, 32
Mata Amritanandamayi, 136
McIver, Wm. J., M.D., 13-14, 17-25, 28-34, 53, 78, 244
metabolism, 27, 129, 150, 220
medical society, 33
medicine (see drugs)
medicine man, 101
medicine teacher, 119
meditation, 11, 40, 69, 102-103, 109, 163, 187, 224, 228, 245, 259, 266
Medjugorje, 71-72
melancholy, 109
Mella, Dorothee, 35, 37, 40, 50, 56, 72, 91, 109, 130, 200, 236, 257
melphalan, 85
memory, 36-37, 59, 62, 91, 144, 232
mental body, 183, 186-187, 189
meridians, 92, 110, 113, 116, 216, 218, 240
messages, 44, 104, 119, 200, 239, 251
metabolism, 27, 129, 150, 220
metastasis, 68
methotrexate, 75
middle world, 190
milk, 109, 118, 158, 204, 207
milk thistle, 158
mind, 10-11, 16, 26, 28, 31, 36, 41, 43, 45-47, 58, 60, 62, 65, 69, 80, 87, 90, 108, 110, 124, 141, 147, 154, 159, 164, 167, 177, 179, 183, 185-187, 193, 198, 207, 211, 218, 223, 225, 227, 232, 247-248, 252-253, 258-260
minerals, 49, 161, 189, 196, 203, 208-209, 214, 231, 238, 240, 267
miracle, 67, 71-72, 96, 250
miracles, 15, 18, 162, 167, 173, 249, 251, 256
Mongoloids, 171-172
Montgomery, 36, 191
mortal oscillatory rate, 220
Moses, Gary L. N.D., 215-218, 223, 228-229
mother, 5, 9, 15-17, 27, 36, 40, 50-51, 53, 55, 59, 67, 69, 71, 79, 88, 98, 103,

work, 8, 16, 27, 33-34, 37-39, 42, 45, 49-51, 66, 68, 84, 96, 99, 103-111, 116, 118-121, 123-127, 136, 141-142, 151, 159, 161, 164, 167, 172-175, 179, 181, 184, 188, 194, 201, 210, 219-220, 225, 228, 230-231, 234-237, 241, 243-246, 248

worth, self, 104, 174, 261

X-Z